ALWAYS MY CHILD

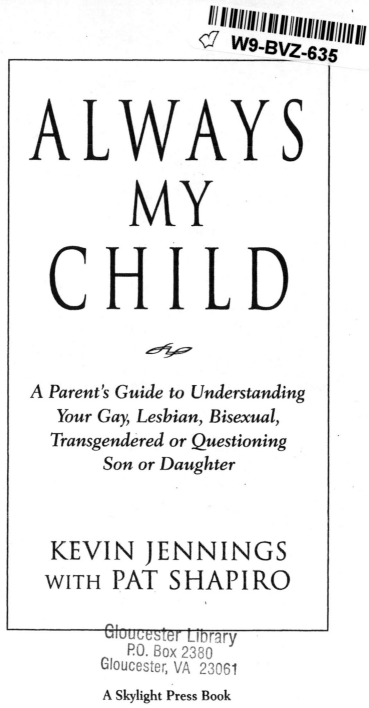

*A Parent's Guide to Understanding
Your Gay, Lesbian, Bisexual,
Transgendered or Questioning
Son or Daughter*

KEVIN JENNINGS
WITH PAT SHAPIRO

A Skylight Press Book
A FIRESIDE BOOK
Published by Simon & Schuster
New York London Toronto Sydney Singapore

FIRESIDE
Rockefeller Center
1230 Avenue of the Americas
New York, NY 10020

For information regarding special discounts for bulk purchases,
please contact Simon & Schuster Special Sales at
1-800-456-6798 or business@simonandschuster.com

Designed by Christine Weathersbee

Manufactured in the United States of America

10   9   8   7   6   5   4   3   2   1

Library of Congress Cataloging-in-Publication Data
Jennings, Kevin, 1963–
    Always my child : a parent's guide to understanding your gay, lesbian,
bisexual, transgendered or questioning son or daughter / Kevin Jennings
with Pat Shapiro.
        p. cm.
    "A Skylight Press book."
    "A Fireside book."
    Includes bibliographical references and index.
    1. Gay teenagers—Social conditions.   2. Gay teenagers—Family
relationships.   3. Parents of gays.   4. Parent and teenager.
I. Shapiro, Patricia Gottlieb.   II. Title.
HQ76.25 .J37   2003
305.235—dc21   2002026785

ISBN 0-7432-2649-6

ACKNOWLEDGMENTS

Always My Child wasn't my idea and I can't take any credit for it! The existence of this book is totally due to the vision of Lynn Sonberg and Meg Schneider, who approached me with the idea, shaped it into a proposal and tirelessly made the rounds of the publishing world until they found a home for it. I cannot thank them enough for their dedication and devotion to this project.

In the "shopping" process, Lynn and Meg could not have found a better champion for *Always My Child* than Doris Cooper of Simon & Schuster. Doris's commitment to this project has been deep and abiding, and she has fought hard every step of the way to make this into the best book possible and to bring it to the widest possible audience. Thank you, Doris, for your support!

The greatest blessing I had in this project has to have been paired with Pat Shapiro as my coauthor. Pat's patience, perseverance and work ethic single-handedly kept the book on schedule and on target. Had Pat not been the coauthor, I can't imagine that this book would ever have seen the light of day. Thank you, Pat, for your kindness, intelligence and commitment!

This project is, ultimately, the outgrowth of my work with GLSEN. The staff, members and supporters of GLSEN must also receive a huge amount of credit for this book. In particular, I'd like to thank: Executive Assistant Liz Carroll, who did invaluable research and made sure that scheduling hurdles were overcome so we stayed on deadline; Student Organizer Chris Tuttle, who leveraged GLSEN's incredible network of more than 1,000 high school–based Gay-Straight Student Alliances to find many of the stories told in the book; and especially Education Director Scott Hirschfeld, who located resources when I needed them, offered important conceptual insights, and did a thorough reading of every page of the manuscript, offering invaluable feedback. Most of all, I'd like to thank our volunteers, our donors, our board, and the grassroots leadership of the organization, which makes its existence possible. I particularly want to thank Charley Todd, Philip Lovejoy and Marty Seldman, who have each been GLSEN's Board President and thus my "boss," which must be one of the toughest jobs on the planet. Your support, guidance and advice have sustained me in this work longer than I thought humanly possible.

This book is built on a foundation of scholarship done by researchers who started work on this subject long before me. I particularly recommend Ritch C. Savin-Williams's *Mom, Dad, I'm Gay* to anyone who wants an in-depth, research-driven understanding of the subject of the dynamics of families with LGBTQ children. Two experts offered invaluable assistance to me directly: Jamison Green, whose interviews in preparation for, and feedback on, the transgender youth chapter are deeply appreciated; and Professor Kevin Kumashiro of Bates College, who offered so many insights in his careful reading and editing of the chapter on LGBTQ youth of color that I must apologize that our limited space did not allow me to capture them all. I recommend his book *Troubling Intersections of Race and Sexuality* for those who wish to examine this important subject in more depth and complexity than a project like *Always My Child* could allow. Thank you. Kevin and Jamison: this book was immeasurably enriched by your contributions.

My mother, Alice Jennings, died just a few days before this book went to press. But my Mom's story (which you will hear about a lot in this book) mirrored the struggles and triumphs many parents of LGBT children go through. I am enormously grateful to her for working through things so that we had the wonderful relationship that we did. Mom, wherever you are, please know that I remain your biggest fan. I am so proud of you, and so proud to be your son.

And my partner Jeff Davis (isn't that a great name for a southern boy to have married?) has exemplified "family values" during our eight years together, constantly supporting me in this difficult work, work that has often landed me at the computer in the wee hours of the morning or in hotel rooms far from home when I should have been with him and our dogs, Luke (1989–2000) and Amber (2000–today). When it comes to family, I am doubly blessed.

—Kevin Jennings

I want to thank my agent, Carol Mann, for recommending me to Meg Schneider and Lynn Sonberg of Skylight Press for this project. I'm grateful to Meg and Lynn for conceiving the idea for this book and for pairing me with Kevin Jennings.

It has been a pleasure to work with Kevin. I owe my education in LGBTQ issues to him. He has been articulate, resourceful and completely supportive.

The drive and passion behind this book has been our editor, Doris Cooper. Throughout the entire process, she never wavered in her commitment to making this book the best possible and has been encouraging, accessible and insightful.

I appreciate the parents and teenagers who spoke to me. They generously shared their experiences because they wanted other parents and teens to know that they were not alone and that they, too, could not only survive their child's coming out but learn and grow as a family from the experience. By allowing me to listen to their pain and their hopes, they expanded my understanding of LGBTQ issues, which, I believe, has made this a richer book.

Lastly, I want to thank my daughter, Margot, my son, Andrew, and my daughter-in-law, Laura, for their encouragement. Most important, I owe a debt of gratitude to my husband, Dick, for his support and patience throughout the challenging process of writing this book while we moved cross country.

—Pat Shapiro

To Judy and Dennis Shepard, Leslie Sadasivan,
Becky and John Glezen, Mary Jane Karger,
Dave and Ruth Waterbury and the thousands
of parents I've met who are working to provide
a better, safer world for their LGBT children

And to the memory of my mother
Alice Johnson Jennings
Nov. 17, 1925–Aug. 17, 2002
For, as Abraham Lincoln once said,
"All that I am or hope to be I owe to
my angel mother."

CONTENTS

INTRODUCTION

When I was growing up in rural North Carolina in the 1970s, I honestly thought I would grow up to be President. After all, that was my birthright as an American. I lived in a country where anyone who was determined and worked hard enough could aspire to the highest office in the land. I planned to live out that American dream.

However, from an early age, I realized that something was amiss.

I knew I was gay long before I had heard that word or knew what it meant. I remember at age six or seven being more fascinated by my brother's bodybuilding magazines than by his *Playboys*, but somehow knowing that this was information I should keep quiet. As I grew up and came to understand what these feelings meant, I recoiled in horror from myself.

Being a boy who loved books and who shied away from grade school machismo—a boy who didn't always conform to the gender expectations of my small-town world—cast me out. By middle school, my classmates had labeled me the "school fag."

The relentless taunting was cruel and soul-destroying. I began to hide in the library during any unstructured time in the school day so I wouldn't be beaten up. I'd eat lunch alone in the hallway to avoid cafeteria teasing. I'd spend every Sunday night battling my "Sunday funny feeling"—a euphemism for the fear-inspired nausea that the prospect of returning to school on Mondays always brought.

When my family moved to another small southern town in 1979, after my sophomore year, I started in a new school and decided to shed my unfortunate past. I pursued what I thought was "normal" with a vengeance. I dated every girl I could literally get my hands on, earning a well-deserved reputation as a big jerk who always tried to see how far he could get on the first date. I was the biggest teller of fag jokes and ridiculed anyone who suggested anything decent about gay people.

What I really hated was myself, and this I could not escape from, regardless of how often I got drunk or stoned, no matter how deeply I retreated into music or magazines, soaking up hours behind the locked door of my bedroom.

I never told my mom that I ate lunch alone everyday. I never revealed that my insides felt chipped away by meanness and alienation. I never let on that I thought I would never fit in anywhere. Only once, did I test the waters. I told her that I was gay and then quickly denied that it was true. That's a common thing LGBT people do. You kind of come out like a turtle, look around to see if it's safe. If it's not, you stick your head back in and scurry away.

The most important thing in my world was making my mother proud; I couldn't—I wouldn't—risk letting her down.

So I bore the burden of my secret shame alone, wondering if my loneliness would ever abate.

YOU KNOW WHAT TO DO

If your child is LGBTQ (lesbian, gay, bisexual, transgender or questioning—terms we'll define later) her day-to-day experience probably mirrors what mine was. While it's true for many LGBTQ youth that there's an unprecedented level of acceptance and support, it is also true that these remain extraordinarily difficult times for young LGBTQ people.

And, like me, I bet one of the most important things for your child is pleasing you—even when you feel like a mere blip cn his or her radar.

If you are one of the millions of parents who suspect that your child is LGBTQ, or if she has just come out to you, you're probably experiencing a kaleidoscope of emotions. Chances are you have burning questions: will my child be okay? Is it my fault? Can I still be a good parent when I don't understand this at all? What am I supposed to do?

We'll cover the emotions later in the book, but for now, I want to get to your questions, so that you can relax a little.

With your support, your child will be just fine.

No, it is not your fault. It is no one's fault.

If you know how to be a good parent—and you do—you know how to serve your LGBTQ child, because she wants the same things that every child wants: to be loved and accepted for who she is.

There is nothing that you are supposed to do that you haven't done before. This book will teach you how to use what you already know. A lot of it is intuitive.

Trust your intuition.

While there is information in this book that may be new to you, you will be applying the skills and techniques that you've used throughout your life as a parent. These are the same skills that you used when you wanted to convey something important to your child from the time she was a toddler: don't touch the stove, don't get into a car with a stranger. Those skills will be applied to situations concerning your child being LGBTQ.

If your child has recently come out, she may no longer feel sure you still love her as much as you did before. She may doubt that you still think she's great. She doesn't automatically assume you still value her for being a star volleyball player or a triumphant student. She probably questions whether you understand what she's going through or if you have any useful guidance to offer. She may think now that all you can see is her sexuality.

So, you need to tell her clearly and often: "I love you. I think you're great. And we'll work together to overcome any challenges you face—just like we always have." You know how to do this. You've done it for years. You make the message clear and you repeat it constantly.

It's straightforward. It's simple. And it works.

"Easier said than done," you're thinking?

Fair enough. Many parents of LGBTQ children feel that they don't know them anymore. Many have qualms and disappointments about having an LGBTQ child. Some sense a rift the size of the Grand Canyon. The trick is to not beat yourself up, to not feel defeated before you've given yourself the opportunity to grow closer to your child, which you can do, just like other parents of LGBTQ children already have. (And some of the most unlikely parents.) *Always My Child* will lend a hand.

Straight parents can't be blamed for not knowing how to proceed when they learn they have an LGBTQ child. You don't know how because you've never been in the position your child is in. In any of the other "minorities" in the United States—people of color or non-Christians like Jews or Muslims, for example—youths usually grow up with parents who are like them. When their children meet discrimination or prejudice, they can turn to their parents, who have probably shared their experiences, and receive empathy and advice. A parent can say, "There's nothing wrong with you. Be proud of who you are, just like I am." Understandably, a straight parent cannot offer the same perspective to her LGBTQ child because she'd had a different life experience. But you can learn. *Always My Child* is designed to help you do so.

Always My Child will also help you move to the next level of developing a strong relationship with your child. The most effective way to do that is to understand the worlds through which she moves in the course of a day, from the classroom to the bagel shop down the street; from your kitchen table to the record store where she works after school.

When you glimpse the contours of your child's sphere, you will begin truly to comprehend what she faces everyday, and giving her the support she needs will come naturally. This book, in turn, will give you guidelines for supporting her in every phase: at home with your family, at school, with her peers, and in the community.

I want to help you in recognizing all of your child's facets so that you see her for more than her sexual identity: you see her as a human being. And, I will show you how to support her so that she never feels alone.

GENDER STRAITJACKETS

To understand what your child is going through every day, we need to step back and take a bird's-eye view of society. For starters, like so many of my straight friends, you may not have realized that our culture is built around a subtle, but pervasive bias, in which the people who make up cultural institutions, such as schools and churches, and even the shops and markets we frequent, are conditioned to expect others to live and behave as if everyone were heterosexual. The first thing parents need to recognize—which is almost impossible to see unless it is pointed out to them—is that there is a pervasive societal idea that everyone is straight unless proven otherwise.

And that straight is better than LGBTQ.

This message, with its stereotypes and innuendos, reverberates within every LGBTQ young person. Like an incessant jackhammer outside the window, the notion that there is something wrong—abnormal—follows LGBTQ youth everywhere they go . . . and often all the way home.

When I reflect on my junior high school years now, I see how the ridicule and harassment that I blamed on my peers stemmed from the stereotypes and myths that suffuse our culture. Not that the kids who tormented me were blameless. Not at all. But kids don't like anything that deviates from "the norm." And they learn that norm from society's signals and cultural myths at a very early age: in the toys they play with, the colors they wear, the television shows they watch and the way they act in school and on the playground. Some messages are blatant, while others seamlessly invade our culture through religion, the media and yes, our very own families.

Recently we've seen tremendous change in attitudes to sexuality, sexual orientation and gender identification. In such a rapidly changing world, young people—both heterosexual and homosexual—are uncertain how to behave. With many floundering and looking for something familiar they can rely on, they succumb to the intense pressure from peers to squeeze themselves into what I call gender straitjackets: prescribed, stereotypical notions of what is acceptable male and female behavior.

Boys feel pressure to act macho, be tough and flaunt their dates with girls. Any deviation—a talent in dramatic

Young people today receive enormously conflicting messages around sexual orientation. There is much more social acceptance of LGBTQ people, but also much more violence and harassment as they become more visible. Young people are coming out at younger ages while their peers may feel more and more hostile to the increasingly visible LGBTQ community in their midst because, for the first time, straight children have to confront their prejudices and deep-seated fears. There is a tremendous irony here, but it is the reality: there is much greater visibility and support for LGBTQ young people, and yet they are a bigger target than in the past.

arts or a preference for dance—brings a social penalty: they are swiftly labeled "gay" because these (and other) interests have been stereotyped as "girl" activities. Girls, too, must play a traditional part: looking and acting feminine and dating guys. They have a little more leeway than boys (girls can wear "boy" clothes like jeans), but if they are too interested in sports, don't wear makeup or show little interest in "putting out" for boys, their peers call them "dykes."

Why is homosexuality so troubling to many Americans? One reason that some people feel uncomfortable with LGBTQ people is because of the "sex" in homosexuality. In fact, that may have been the first thing you thought of when you learned your child was LGBTQ: What does he do with his friends? How does she experience pleasure? In this country, we tend to define homosexuals by their sexual behavior. We don't see heterosexuals in the same way. We see heterosexuals as people first and define them by their roles or occupations: lawyer, nurse, social worker, mother, brother. The fact that they are attracted to the opposite sex is not their defining characteristic. With time, you will be able to see your child in this broader way too.

As co-founder and executive director of Gay, Lesbian, Straight Education Network, known as GLSEN, the largest organization in the United States whose mission is to make schools safe for LGBTQ youth, I've worked with schools and communities in forty-four states on LGBTQ issues. I have encountered school principals and teachers who both wittingly and unwittingly perpetrate stereotypes. I have met well-meaning school board members who believe that an LGBTQ child who's been victimized should simply change schools but don't realize that it is the schools that need to change. I have talked to wonderful, involved, loving parents who don't notice that their child's unhappiness comes from a silent source of shame. While talking to these myriad people, I have been able to put my finger on the pulse of America and I have seen, firsthand, the way our culture and its expectations shape the real life day-to-day struggles of LGBTQ children and their families.

It's important for parents to recognize cultural myths so that they don't perpetuate stereotypes in raising their families. That's not always easy to do, however, because many parents actually want their children to fit the traditional mold. These parents are more comfortable with a conventional, conforming child who validates their lifestyle.

But this is generally not what is best for your child.

ALWAYS YOUR CHILD

When teens come out, they often question their place in their family, their school, their religion, and their community, and wonder if they still belong to any of these critical institutions. That's one of the reasons it's important for you to understand your child and her world: She needs to know she is still loved and still belongs.

While many LGBTQ youth fit in well everywhere and have a dynamism that energizes their friends and family, there are LGBTQ youth who, like me years ago, withdrew from everyone and everything, especially themselves. Adolescents today have greater knowledge, more information, and more diverse sexual experiences than previous generations. They are having sex earlier, more often and with more partners. They face social and interpersonal situations in high school that I would imagine you barely touched in your twenties. Yet, there's a paradox: today's youth are more isolated from one another and from their families and schools than any other generation. This is especially true for LGBTQ youth.

Throughout this book, I'm going to talk about the importance of young people developing a healthy identity that is consistent

with who they are inside. One way to do that is to help them connect with other people, both their own age and older, who share
their sexual orientation so they can understand they are not
alone and that they are not freaks.

There is an important reason for doing this: isolated teens are
at risk. If young people don't feel that sense of connection,
chances are they are going to get in trouble. They may drink ex-
cessively and do drugs. They may develop an eating disorder.
They may fail to protect themselves from pregnancy, sexually
transmitted diseases and AIDS. Why should they behave differently? No one seems to care.

Yet, what convinces them otherwise isn't anything fancy. Like
me, they simply want their parents' unconditional love and support, and to know that they haven't disappointed you. They want
to hear, "You are always my child."

This book is designed to help the growing number of parents
who either want to stand with their child, advocate for her, and
help her connect to family members, friends, and special communities, or to at least get themselves to the point where they
can better understand her.

A NEW GENERATION OF PARENTS

Times are changing for parents, too. One of the shifts I've seen
over the seventeen years I've worked on LGBT issues is a real
evolution in the attitudes of many parents. I first observed this
about four or five years ago at the GLSEN Pathfinder Annual
Awards, which honor students, teachers or parents for outstand-
ing achievement in ending anti-LGBT bigotry. For many years,
the students who won our top awards would come alone or with
their friends. About three or four years ago, I noticed their parents were suddenly there, beaming.

I began to note who this new generation of parents was; even if they were having trouble accepting their child, they were beginning to play a role in her life, rather than try to "fix" her.

Part of the reason for the change is that so many of us know LGBTQ people today. According to a 2001 study by the Kaiser Family Foundation, 25 percent of all families say they have a family member who is lesbian, gay or bisexual. A 2001 poll by Lake, Snell, Perry & Associates, a public opinion research firm in Washington, D.C., found that 57 percent of parents say they have a co-worker who is LGBT. Eighty-one percent think children know their sexual orientation by the time they graduate from high school.

LGBTQ people are part of the world for this generation of parents, and they are increasingly prepared to accept and deal with that reality.

More and more, parents have an opportunity to connect with other parents of LGBTQ teens. You need a support network just as much as your child does. There is nothing wrong with reaching out. I'll show you how to take advantage of these opportunities for yourself and how to use them to support your child in doing so.

WHAT THIS BOOK WILL COVER

This guidebook will give you commonsense, plain English explanations of the issues and tell you specifically how to deal with them.

Early in the book, I'll set guidelines for the four essential keys to making your home a safe haven for your teen. They are:

1. Separate your issues from your child's. Discover how to recognize and put aside your own beliefs, prejudices and fears so your child's concerns can take center stage.

2. Get the facts. Find ways to inform yourself about healthy sexual development, safe sex and sexual identity issues.

3. Keep the lines of communication open. Learn when to talk and when to keep silent as well as specific techniques, such as when and how to follow up on a child's hint about sexual orientation or gender identity.

4. Create an open atmosphere. Learn specific ways to create a home that reflects tolerance for diversity.

I'll also guide you step-by-step through:

- your child's coming-out process
- the stages of your own process of acceptance
- your child's challenges at school with her peers and teachers
- advocating for your child at school
- ensuring safety on the Internet
- recognizing signs of serious trouble

Each chapter will contain specific dialogues so you know exactly what to say and when to say it. These dialogues include examples showing you what to say:

- to encourage your child to be honest with you
- to help your child break the ice and come out to you
- to tell your child's grandparent she's LGBTQ
- to help your child stand up to bullies
- to express your concern if you recognize the warning signs of a serious problem developing

The key to a happy family—and happy children—is the parent. Your family is the primary source of your child's self-acceptance and self-esteem. A parent's approval signals to a child that she is loved, valued and accepted. Every child wants these things, but few worry about them as intensely as children who are LGBTQ. After all, few issues are as central to teenagers' self-esteem as how they feel about their sexual selves. Feeling good about one's sexual identity is one of the most critical challenges of adolescence. And the odds are against that happening easily for LGBTQ young people in today's society.

All the research shows that the need for affirmation from parents grows more intense as children become teenagers. Adolescence is a time of healthy and exciting exploration: Who am I? What are my true interests? What makes me happy? These are questions teens must answer. Consistent acceptance and support at home is the best way for them to investigate these issues and to begin to draw some conclusions.

I hope that reading this book will be one step in the process by which you come to be able to fully embrace your LGBTQ child, help ease tensions at home, and enable you to be the kind of parent you want to be.

AUTHORS' NOTE

We will alternate by chapter between using masculine and feminine pronouns to refer to LGBTQ youth throughout the book.

We have changed the names of students and parents, who are identified by first name only, to protect their privacy. Some of their identifying information has also been modified. If someone is called by their first and last name, that name has not been changed.

The term "parents" should be read to include all caretakers, including guardians and other family members in a parenting role.

Finally, this book is particularly unusual because it explores three other issues that most other parenting books don't discuss: the concerns unique to transgender teens, questioning teens and teens of color. Each of these groups has special needs and deserves focused attention, which we have done by giving each its own chapter.

Chapter One

YOU AND YOUR TEEN

Understanding Your Issues,
Making Your Home a Safe Harbor

THE COURSE OF YOUR child's future may seem different from what you envisioned, but he is the same person he
was before he told you he was LGBTQ. Nothing has changed except that you now know that he is attracted to someone of the
same gender.

The things you loved about him have not changed. If you
loved his quirky sense of humor, it's still there. If you were proud
of her thoughtfulness, she's just as considerate now. Your child's
path in life may now be different than you expected it to be, but
his character is the same.

Character is not defined by what you are but by who you are:
Are you hard working? Do you treat other people respectfully?
Do you have integrity? These qualities do not change because
your child comes out, but some parents have a tendency to obscure positive character traits in the coming-out process.

I know my parents did. After my father "found Jesus" in the
early 1950s, he devoted the remaining twenty years of his life to
bringing the gospel to others. My religious upbringing as a
Southern Baptist taught me that homosexuals were perverts des-
tined for eternal damnation.

When I was a child, fear ruled my world. Having realized that

I was gay from an early age, I grew up terrified of the lake of fire in which I would burn for eternity because of my "unnatural desires." But worse than the fear of eternal damnation was the prospect of Judgment Day. Even though I'd had no sexual experiences yet, I was terrified because of the Baptist belief that wanting to do something was as sinful as actually doing it. The transgressions of one junior high gym class seemed enough to keep God busy for hours: "At 9:30 and 22 seconds, had lustful thoughts about Todd Burton. At 9:30 and 27 seconds, coveted Mike Visone. At 9:30 and 34 seconds, longed for Tripp Winston" and so on. Of course, I didn't share these wicked thoughts with a soul.

Your child, too, has thoughts, fears and experiences at school that you and others may not know about. He may have to contend with friends he feels he has let down or disappointed. His peers may have envisioned his future differently, as you have. Now they may turn on him or taunt him, even though he may not feel that he's changed.

I did not come out until I had moved far enough away from home to feel safe to do so. But I often think back about how different my life would have been if I had been raised in an open, accepting atmosphere. In school I was tormented, teased and beaten. But I never felt I could come home to tell my family why this was happening to me or ask them for help.

Home should be the one place where every child feels safe: where he belongs and basks in love, where he knows he is understood and accepted, whether he's a quarterback poet, she's a young lesbian, or they are struggling to figure out their sexual orientation. Most parents desire this atmosphere for their children; they know that children prosper in a warm, loving home.

But *desiring* it and *creating* it are two different things.

Communication, the key to all healthy relationships, is also crucial to achieving this kind of home. Throughout the book, I'll guide you in initiating conversations with your child and show you how to talk to him about the various stages of coming out, and your own process of moving toward acceptance.

Young people thrive when they have a knowledgeable adult—ideally a parent—as their source of information and support. When they feel they can't talk to their parent or be themselves, they can feel alienated and misunderstood. They may try to get attention by letting their grades falter, skipping classes or losing interest in subjects they once excelled in. Alienated children often become troubled children: they strike out in anger, clash with the law, or withdraw into a shell. These crises can be prevented. That is your challenge.

From my workshops with parents and my lectures and involvement with teenagers in schools across the country, I've learned what it takes to make your home a safe harbor for your child. You may have your own definition of a safe harbor, based on your own upbringing, your values and your ideas. What you bring to this process sets the groundwork for what I'm going to tell you.

In this chapter, I'll introduce the four essential keys to making your home safe for your teen. I'll set the guidelines for each of these keys here and refer to them throughout the book. Keep in mind that these are not presented in chronological order. Each is equally important. You will probably do them all simultaneously. They are:

1. Separate your issues from your child's

2. Get the facts

3. Keep the lines of communication open

4. Create an open atmosphere

SEPARATE YOUR ISSUES
FROM YOUR CHILD'S

The first step towards supporting your child is facing your own assumptions about sexual diversity, because your attitudes pervade the home and set the tone. You may still have prejudices, but once you've committed to managing them so that you can be an effective parent to your child, you will be better able to develop an open atmosphere at home for your teenager. Then you will be able to discuss critical issues, such as sexual and emotional health, clearly, comfortably, and in detail. That may sound scary to you right now, but I'll guide you through the process.

One word of warning: Don't expect your child to help you resolve your issues. He has too much going on himself. There's a fine line here: It's important to let your child know you are working on your attitudes, but at the same time, don't expect him to walk you through every phase. This is a very individual process. You will have to gauge how much you share against how receptive your child is to being included in your struggle. We will discuss this in more detail in Chapter 5.

There is a very good reason for developing an open atmosphere at home: If your child feels strong and self-caring, he is less likely to behave recklessly sexually. And, he will want you to be a part of his life, which will give you the chance to pass your values on to your child.

Stuart, a sixteen-year-old straight boy, approached me when I spoke at his school and told me, "In middle school I wanted to be a ballet dancer, but my dad said, 'You can't do ballet. That's what fags do.'" In high school, Stuart wanted to join the chorus, but his dad told him, "You can't be in the chorus, that's for queers." With great sadness, Stuart said to me, "My dad is taking everything good out of my life."

Stuart was despondent because he could not pursue his passions. As he gets older, he may defy his father's wishes and pursue them anyhow. But no doubt, his father's negative comments will continue to dampen his spirit and may possibly build a wall between them—whatever he decides to do.

Sadly, Stuart's father may not even be aware of what he is doing, because he is operating from his own unconscious belief system.

Self-Reflection

There may be times when you don't feel like being the supportive parent, when you just wish this whole issue would go away. That's natural. But this issue is not going to disappear. Much as you may hope that your child is going through a phase, most likely, he is not.

Your conscious and unconscious motivations and expectations about sexual identity affect your parenting an LBGTQ child.

Try to carve out a block of time in your day when you won't be disturbed to explore the following questions. Take time to think about each one. Don't gloss over them. You may want to get out a notebook and pen and keep a journal. When you write your responses, rather than just think about them, you give each question deeper consideration.

Close your eyes and remember when your child was first born. Think about your expectations as a parent and about everything you hoped for and wanted for your child's life. Explore the following questions:

- What motivated you to have children?
- What qualities did you think you needed to have to be a good parent?
- How did you visualize your child's adult life? Was it like yours? If not, how was it different?
- What profession did you think your child would have?
- What interests or hobbies?
- Did you see your child marrying and having children?
- Did you anticipate having grandchildren?
- What were your goals for your children?

Once you have answered these questions thoroughly, take a break of a few hours or a day and then set aside another block of time to explore the following questions about sexual identity.

The first few questions focus on your own sexual identity. The remaining ones will help you examine your attitudes toward people who are LGBTQ. Again, give yourself plenty of time for reflection and try to write your answers down. Use these questions as a springboard:

- When did you become aware that you were attracted to boys or girls or both?
- How did you feel about that?
- How did your family and community react to that realization?
- How did your religious and cultural traditions support you?
- When were you first aware that there were LGBTQ people in the world?
- Was your first impression negative or positive?
- What kind of things have you heard about LGBTQ people since then?
- What have been your contacts with LGBTQ people, either personally or in the news, movies or television?

After you have taken the time to answer both sets of questions, then put the two scripts together and think about how the first script would change if you had a LGBTQ child. For example, if your idea of a good parent was someone who was nurturing and loved her child unconditionally, how would that change if your son were LGBTQ? Or if you visualized your daughter replicating your life and giving you grandchildren, how would you feel if she were a lesbian?

For some parents, the formation of traditional families is the basis of their sense of identity and self-worth. When things don't go according to the ingrained heterosexist script, it may threaten their whole sense of being. It causes them to question themselves and ask: Where did I go wrong?

A Parent's Expectations

The fact that your child is LGBTQ is not a reflection of you, your lifestyle, your parenting skills, or your masculinity or femininity. While no one is absolutely sure what causes homosexuality, the American Psychiatric Association, for example, believes that innate characteristics contribute to sexual orientation and that orientation cannot be changed through medical or psychiatric treatment. Homosexuality is not caused by something a parent does. Yet many parents, on first learning their child is LGBTQ, feel that they must have done something wrong to cause his homosexuality.

Anne recalls how she reacted when she found out her daughter was a lesbian. "Never for a moment did I think that I wasn't going to love her, support her or care about her. None of that. Just a terrible disappointment that the hopes and dreams and expectations that I wanted for my child . . ." her voice trails off as a sadness creeps in. How did she visualize her daughter's life? "With a lovely career that would very much be a part of her life, but that she would also get married, have children, and have a white picket fence to boot."

Anne's vision for her daughter was an outgrowth of her own value system and expectations. Parents who hope their children will continue the family name and produce grandchildren may be threatened by a life that doesn't automatically lead to forming another heterosexual family. It feels like an indictment of their own choices. Mothers, in particular, often ask their LGBTQ children: "How could you possibly be happy?" The implication in their question is that a life like theirs is the key to happiness. Even though many LGBTQ people do become parents, some mothers (and fathers) fixate on the potential loss of grandchildren when their own child first comes out.

If their son turns out to be gay, many fathers feel as though they failed as a dad to impart good masculine values. They see their son as a mirror of their own masculinity and their own choices in life. This is a perfectly natural reaction.

The situation is even more complicated in divorced families. When the mother has custody, the father often feels angry when their son turns out to be gay. On some level, the father believes that if he had stayed with his wife, their son would have had a masculine influence and wouldn't be gay.

Political Beliefs

Parents with a higher level of awareness on LGBTQ issues do tend to be more accepting of their child more quickly than those who do not, but there are far too many painful exceptions to this rule. Parenting is not about your political beliefs or your religious beliefs. It is an outgrowth of your own identity, your values and expectations, and your particular life path.

Your initial reaction to the fact that you have an LGBTQ child usually grows out of your own value system and expectations. It can have surprisingly little to do with your political beliefs. Many children grow up in educated, liberal homes, yet their parents still have difficulty when they learn their child is LGBTQ. Conversely, some deeply conservative parents set aside their conventional beliefs to stand by their child.

Joni's parents were activists. They marched for abortion rights and gay pride, and discussed left-wing causes at the dinner table. Yet, when Joni told them that she thought she was bisexual, her mother vehemently objected: She told her she didn't believe in bisexuality, that deep in her heart she knew Joni was straight, that this was a phase she'd outgrow and that she didn't want to hear any more talk of bisexuality. Her dad was a little more tempered.

Joni recalls, "It was just so scary for me to talk to them about it. They didn't make it something that I felt comfortable talking about, which is really weird because, I feel comfortable talking to them about a ton of stuff and I really love my parents and re-spect them. I'm definitely friends with them as well as having that parent-child relationship, but this issue is something we just don't talk about."

What would she have liked from her parents? Joni replies, "I would have liked to see books around the house about dealing with your gay child. I would like them to have addressed it as a real issue and not something that was mine to deal with, because it was really hard. It was scary.

"It made me sad to see other people's mothers come to diversity conferences with them, and I was wondering, why aren't my parents trying? They're not ignorant people. I wanted them to show some kind of support other than 'Well, we love you no matter what.' I wanted it to be 'We love you and we accept that you're gay and we're not going to overlook that.' "

Joni didn't expect perfection from her parents, or even total understanding. She just wanted a sense that they were making an effort to understand and support her.

Like Joni, children of liberal parents are often shocked and disappointed at their parents' reaction. Chastity Bono, Sonny Bono and Cher's daughter, sensed her mother's deep disapproval. She writes in her memoir *Family Outing*: "And despite my mother's accepting attitude toward her friends who were gay, I still had a feeling that she didn't want *me* to be gay. I didn't have to be told explicitly; her continued criticism of my tomboyishness felt like a disapproval of my emerging sexuality. As a result, talking to either of my parents about the 'gay issue' seemed out of the question."

As parents we all have an idea, a fantasy, of what our children's lives will be like. Yet very rarely do their destinies end up plugging into that. Some parents want their children to be doctors or teachers. Some fantasize about a child who makes the world a better place. Regardless, children develop to a certain extent independent of their parents, and independent of their wishes.

That's why it's tough even for liberal parents to accept an LGBTQ child. It's a surprise, and parents (like most humans) generally don't like surprises.

Moral Issues

If you believe that being LGBTQ is morally wrong, you have a very difficult task ahead of you. We all have grown up with belief systems that help us make sense of the world. Now, suddenly, your child is challenging yours.

I must tell you that it will be difficult for you to hold on to everything you have believed to date, and still have a warm, positive relationship with your child. At the same time, keep in mind that you do not have to abandon all your religious or cultural beliefs either. For a lot of people, it's scary to see their religious beliefs threatened, because beliefs give meaning to their lives.

Give yourself some time and space to explore your beliefs with the new knowledge you have about your child. I understand that this is asking a lot because these beliefs are core to you and how you understand the world.

Basically you have three choices:

1. Abandon your beliefs totally.

   This is probably not a realistic choice for most people because religious beliefs are strongly ingrained from a young age. You would probably feel as though you had lost your anchor if you discarded your beliefs totally, and might feel resentful toward your child for "pushing" in this direction.

2. Stick rigidly to your religious beliefs.

   If you choose your moral or religious beliefs over your child, you have to understand that this will inevitably lead to conflict with your child and impair your ability to support him. It may sound harsh, but in the end, parents with deeply held anti-LGBT beliefs are going to have a hard time, and we cannot deny it. If you say something such as, "You're my child but I think homosexuality is wrong. It's not what God wants for you," you will drive your child away. He'll either drop out of your life, because, in the end, that message is just too painful to hear, or he will engage in self-destructive behavior because he believes your negative message is right.

If you choose this route, then you have to ask yourself if that's the end of the script you wanted for your parenting—having your child absent from your life in any meaningful way?

I'm advocating that you rethink some of your attitudes and put your child's health and well-being ahead of your own moral or religious beliefs. If you don't, you will lose your child, because he will feel judged, rather than valued, loved and accepted.

3. Find a way to hold on to the parts of your religion that you believe in most strongly, while integrating acceptance of your child to create a new understanding.

Integration may not be possible in all religious traditions because of their strict rules, but for many people, this is the most sensible way to handle the conflict.

This was an issue I struggled with personally. Raised by a Southern Baptist evangelist, I went to church every Sunday morning, Sunday night and Wednesday night of my childhood. I memorized thousands of Bible verses. For a long time, I felt that my being gay had precluded my being religious.

As an adult, however, I thought about what the central messages—not the rules—of the teachings I grew up with were. I discarded a lot of the literal interpretations of the Bible and kept the central message: Do unto others as you would have them do unto you. Within that context, I decided that homophobia was sinful, not homosexuality. If I didn't want to be a victim of prejudice, I shouldn't visit prejudice on someone else. With time, I came to understand the work I do now as an outgrowth of the religious teachings I was raised with.

Here's another idea that may help you look at your beliefs in a new way: Say that your idea of a good parent is someone who gives unconditional love and is always there for her child. Then, I would ask you to make those values the primary ones that guide how you interact with your child. In other words, if you believe your child needs unconditional love, acceptance and support, then use that as the filter through which you pass everything you say, rather than your religious beliefs.

You may have to make some choices about when and how you express your religious beliefs. Before you speak, ask yourself: What is more important to me, the moral or religious beliefs I hold or the health and well-being of my child?

GET THE FACTS

Your child probably knew that he was LGBTQ for three to four years before he came out to you. That means he's much more comfortable with and knowledgeable about the subject than you are. Let him be your guide and suggest readings that would be helpful, meetings to attend and other resources. If you are concerned that he's asking you to do too much too soon, Chapter 5 will offer suggestions on handling this.

TIP: Check the Resources Section at the back of the book for faith-based LGBTQ groups, where you can meet others who have reconciled their religious beliefs with LGBTQ issues.

I suggest that you begin a

parallel process of obtaining information by investigating a number of areas, while you continue to explore your own beliefs, history and biases. The following issues are good places to begin. They are also covered in this book:

- the difference between orientation, behavior and identity (Chapter 2)
- the typical coming-out process (Chapter 5)
- the conditions LGBTQ students face in schools and elsewhere, and the impact of this hostility on their physical and mental health (Chapters 4, 9, 10)
- up-to-the-minute facts on safe sexual health (Chapter 2)
- Internet safety (Chapter 5)
- information on your child's legal rights (Appendix)

Having misinformation or the wrong information perpetuates stereotypes. Being grounded in facts will help you feel less uncomfortable or embarrassed when you have discussions with your child. In addition, at some point, you may be in a position to help educate family members and friends.

Once you have zeroed in on the kinds of information you need, explore the Resources section at the back of the book. These sources will be invaluable to you.

KEEP THE LINES OF
COMMUNICATION OPEN

You're probably familiar with this dialogue: Your fifteen-year-old son comes home from school and you greet him:

"How was school?"

"Fine."

"What'd you do today?"

"Nothing."

He grabs a snack and heads to his room, not to be seen or heard from until dinner. Such interactions are frustrating. You mean well, you're there and ready to talk, and he has nothing to say—to you.

It's not uncommon for teenagers to brush off their parents. Parents then shy away from communication because they don't want to be rejected by their children. That's a natural reaction, but it doesn't help to create open communication.

Your attempts at conversation may not always go smoothly. You can do everything right and still be rebuffed. Of course, you want to engage your child, but he may not be ready to talk. The important thing is that you are trying. You are sending him signals that you are interested. He will remember this and come back to talk when he's ready.

Rejection is also a huge issue for your LGBTQ teen. Many purposely distance themselves from their parents and keep their thoughts and feelings close to their vests because they fear you will reject them for being LGBTQ.

Here are some general guidelines for opening the channels of communication in your home, and some specific ones for talking about issues that concern your LGBTQ child.

Be Ready to Listen

There's an old dictum for social workers: Begin where the client is. The same is true for parents: Begin where your child is. One parent complained that her son always brushed her off when she questioned him about his day when he walked in from school, but at ten o'clock at night, after he finished his homework, he'd come down to the den and talk nonstop. She was exhausted and could hardly keep her eyes open. But because he wanted to talk, she listened. And she learned a lot.

Your child will not talk when *you* are ready, but when he is. If he starts talking while you're balancing your checkbook or in the midst of chopping vegetables, do the following:

- Stop what you're doing.
- Look at him and give him your undivided attention.
- If you honestly cannot listen at that moment, explain why and ask if you can talk again at another time.

If you let these times pass or don't pick up on what he says, not only will you miss an opportunity to connect with your child, but he'll be less likely to approach you in the future because he will think you're not accessible.

On the other hand, be aware that your child may be testing you. He knows on some level that he is choosing an awkward moment and may want to make sure that he is your priority. This can be frustrating for a parent, but hang in there. You'll get through the aggravation.

Keep Talking

It's important to keep a dialogue—any dialogue—going with your child. It doesn't have to be about anything in particular. In fact, the less sensitive, the better. The following subjects are non-threatening:

- the movies
- television shows
- your pet
- your relatives

Try to find common ground and keep talking.

David was a quiet fifteen-year-old who shared little of his life with his parents. Two- or three-word answers were his usual reply. But whenever his mother mentioned something about

Honey, the family's cocker spaniel, he came to life and chatted nonchalantly. Once he got going, he often launched into talking about school.

Once your child begins to move into more personal areas, keep in mind that certain words stop a conversation in its tracks. Try to avoid using the following words. What they convey to a teen is in parenthesis:

- "Why don't you?" (advising)
- "Do you realize . . . ? " (lecturing)
- "What you need is . . ." (diagnosing)
- "You should, you ought to . . ." (moralizing)

When your child talks, try to listen between the lines. Joey walked in, threw his book bag on the floor and complained, "My coach is such a bastard." Rather than asking what happened, his father said, "I don't want to hear that word in this house." His reprimand cut off any further conversation. He'll never learn what Joey was so upset about.

Fathers often complain that their children don't tell them anything, that they confide more in their mothers. Part of the reason is that mothers, generally, tend to be around more and do more chatting. This creates a comfort level that some kids don't experience with their fathers. When children are ready to open up, they're going to talk to the parent who they feel is more accepting and with whom they feel most comfortable.

If you're a dad, make an attempt to talk more with your child about school. Begin a dialogue by asking every day, "Tell me about your day," then apply the listening skills that follow. Try not to ask questions that can be answered with "yes" or "no." Be aware of your tendency to reply, "Ask your mother" when a child asks you a question. Instead, give his question full consideration. You can then say, "Your mother and I will discuss it." Also notice whether you go to your wife with a question about your child ("How did Jimmy do on his test?"), rather than speaking to him directly. If you catch yourself doing this, begin talking to him face-to-face, rather than using your wife as an intermediary.

Timing Matters

It's often easier to talk while you're doing something else. The conversation can seem more casual and your child may be more relaxed because he doesn't feel as if he's in the hot seat. For those very reasons, these conversations are often more meaningful than when you sit your child down and say, "We need to talk." Those words are sure to clam him up or put him on the defensive.

Try chatting while cooking dinner, gardening, or reading the Sunday paper. You can initiate a conversation by using the following openers:

- "You know, I've been thinking about something a lot . . ."
- "This is not a big deal, but I'm just curious . . ."
- "Help me out with this. I'm a little confused."

You can also start a conversation by saying, "There's something I'd like to talk to you about. Is this a good time?" Or, you can say, "There's something on my mind. Got a few minutes?" This way you prepare your child that this conversation has a serious nature and may take some time. It's not a conversation you want to have on the fly.

If there are three or four obvious paths the conversations might take and two of them make you very uncomfortable, then don't even begin the conversation. If you're not going to be happy to learn your child is LGBTQ, you shouldn't initiate the conversation until you can work through your feelings. Given the fear of rejection that many LBGTQ youth bring to the issue of disclosure, saying the wrong thing in the beginning may cause them to pull back for good.

Teens also leave hints that they want to talk. If your daughter leaves her journal on the coffee table and it's usually hidden up in her room, you can say, "I noticed that your journal was left downstairs last night. You don't usually do that." And go wherever the conversation takes you.

Driving in the car is also a good time to talk because you have a captive audience. Cheryl, the mother of a teenage girl, found that when she drove carpool after soccer practice she learned a lot. She listened unobtrusively when the girls talked and after she dropped off the last girl, would often raise a question about something that had been said. Her daughter, who was in a relaxed, chatty mood, seemed more receptive to talking than at home where she accused her mother of being too intrusive.

Just Listen

Teenagers say the biggest mistake their parents make when discussing sex is that they spend too much time preaching and too little time listening, Dr. Nathalie Bartle, author of *Venus in Blue Jeans,* told *The New York Times.* [*]

Indeed, keeping still is one of the most difficult tasks for parents. That means: no nagging, criticizing, lecturing, giving advice unless asked, not barraging them with questions, and letting them talk without interrupting.

Responses that encourage your child to talk and show that you're listening include:

> "Tell me more about that."
> "How do you feel about that?"
> "Really? That's interesting."

[*] Gilbert, Susan, "Teaching Teenagers a Subject Many Know All Too Well," *The New York Times,* October 10, 2000, p. F7.

When you listen, be aware of the following body language:

- Sitting with your arms crossed creates a barrier and makes you appear angry.
- Nodding from time to time shows that you're listening.
- Maintaining eye contact means you're connecting.

Broach Sensitive Subjects Sensitively

It's never too late to start talking to your teenager.

Bring up a sensitive subject by leading into it gradually. Consider using an article in the newspaper or an incident from a movie or television show as a springboard for discussion. Let's say you noticed that your daughter has started hanging out with a different group of girls and you think they might be lesbians. You thought your daughter was straight but now you're not sure. One way to broach the subject is to watch *Will and Grace* with her. After the show, you can ask, "Do you think straight and gay kids can be friends or are there too many differences in their lives?"

See where the discussion leads. If she continues to talk in the abstract, move the discussion into a more personal arena by asking, "What's it like at your school?" If she talks about others at her school, listen and then ask, "What's your experience been?" She may talk about the fact that she's straight and her new girl friends are lesbians and they get along fine, or she may hint that she's unsure of her orientation. Take her comments at face value and reflect on what you hear. You might say, "It sounds like you're questioning your orientation right now," and see where she goes with it. If you sense that she's confused but not ready to talk about it, tell her, "It seems like something's on your mind. When you're ready to talk, I'm here."

Assess Clues Carefully

When Chastity Bono was trying to come out to her dad, she would ask questions such as, "Is there anything I could do that would make you not love me?" She would bring up LGBTQ current events in a casual way, testing to see how he'd respond. One time she left a lesbian romance novel on her nightstand, hoping he'd find it. Eventually, he said to her, "Chas, I've been feeling that you want to talk to me about something." After hemming and hawing, she blurted out, "I'm gay."*

Sometimes, however, you may think you see a clue and it's not one. If you project ideas on to your child, rather than just noting the behavior, it will create problems. When Sam, a straight college student went home for Thanksgiving, his family told homophobic jokes at the dinner table. He put up with it for a while and then said, "I wish you wouldn't say these things because one of my best friends is gay and it's really offensive to me." Everybody stopped talking. That night when he went to bed, his mother came into his room, sat on the edge of his bed, and said, "Sam, I just want to ask you—are you your best friend?" He replied, "No, I was just offended by the jokes." She pressed on, "You can tell me. Are you gay?" Sam insisted, "Mom, I'm not gay."

You have to be careful not to jump to conclusions. If your child chooses to do his seventh-grade debate topic on gay marriage or starts asking questions about how two men have a baby, you must simply meet the child where he is and ask questions in such a way that they open the dialogue.

These may be clues that a child is LGBTQ, but they may not be as well.

Simply note the behavior that has caught your attention. You can say, "I'm really interested that you chose gay marriage as your

* Bono, Chastity, pp. 82–83.

seventh grade term paper topic." And let the child take it where he may. Or, "I see you're curious about how two men have a baby." Let the child respond.

Young people are like firefighters in a burning house. They feel the door and if it's warm, they don't open it, because the fire is on the other side. If the door is cool, they open the door and proceed cautiously. It's not your job to yank the door open and singe your child. It's your job to send signals by noting the clues and then if a child wants to open the door, he will.

Your child will only drop clues for so long. If you don't pick up on them, eventually he will go elsewhere for information—to his peers or the Internet. Your task is to get yourself ready for these conversations: to start thinking and doing some of the exercises I suggested on pages 19–20 so you can handle these discussions with less anxiety.

Frame Discussions in a Health Context, Not a Moral One

Your child is going to get his information from somewhere— that is the reality—and nothing you do can change that. If you have strong religious beliefs that oppose homosexuality, your child will probably see you as judgmental. If he does, he is going to go somewhere else for advice. As discussed earlier, try to temper your beliefs without abandoning them entirely.

Although sexual orientation encompasses more than sexual behavior, most of your discussion will probably center around behavior. If you can, put your religious beliefs aside and try to think about sexual behaviors as either safe or dangerous. Then discuss them from a health viewpoint, not a moral one. Try to make that distinction very clearly to your child, because if you push a moral context, some teens will engage in unsafe sexual behavior just because they've been told it is wrong. It's almost like they are saying, "Watch me do something wrong."

No responsible health professional believes people choose to be LGBT or straight, but all agree there is an element of choice around sexual behavior. If you have strong moral beliefs but want to keep the lines of communication open, I suggest you do two things:

1. Separate your message from a moral judgment around whether your child is LGBTQ or straight. If you believe premarital sex is wrong, it should not matter whether your child is LGBTQ or straight. You might say, "I love you, honey, no matter whether you are gay or straight, but I am concerned about you engaging in sexual behavior of any kind." And then tell him why. Be honest about your values and own them as yours—admitting that they are not necessarily right for everyone else.

2. Explain your position as growing out of your heritage and not as an absolute. You can say to your child, "Right or wrong, when I was growing up there were very different views of LGBTQ people. I'm trying to understand this new world where there are many views of homosexuality. Give me a break as I try and do that."

You have the right and the responsibility to tell your child, "This is what I believe," but the danger here is when you then say, "And this is a universal truth. If you do this, you are going to hell." Then you create a climate where your child becomes terrified and isolated.

If you do believe that particular behaviors are morally wrong, it is pointless to try to pretend something else. That would be inauthentic and children can read that. But you must understand and accept that there is more than one truth. To make your position clear, speak with "I" statements, such as "I feel," or "I think," rather than "This is true." When you speak from "I" statements, you allow that there is more than one truth, which creates an accepting atmosphere and allows the channels of communication to remain open.

CREATE AN OPEN ATMOSPHERE

The major task of adolescence is for teens to establish a sense of who they are. They develop their own identity by experimenting and trying on new roles and behavior in an attempt to differentiate themselves from you. That may take the form of pink hair, a pierced tongue, tattoos, or engaging in activities that are deliberately different from the ones you have favored. Teens want to have a distinct personality, their own likes and dislikes, their unique attitudes. Developing their own identity is what teenagers do and it is perfectly normal.

Your task is three-fold:

1. to give them the space and time to explore options and roles

2. to support their individuality with unconditional love

3. to keep a sense of connectedness to the family so they have a secure base from which to grow.

As young people come into their own physically and emotionally, they may not make the choices you want. But if you love them, regardless of the choices they make, they will grow up with a strong sense of self.

If you are threatened by your child's search to figure out who he is and react with stricter rules or more severe punishment, he may respond by rebelling. If you send a message of shame or disapproval, chances are you will distance your child: being around you will only incite shame.

Aaron knows what that feels like. He is a college student whose parents know he's gay, but they rarely talk about it. He says, "Usually, when I come home for a vacation they'll try to bring it up. First they'll ask me if I'm still gay and I'll say 'yes,' and they'll want me to see some psychiatrist. Sometimes we fight. Eventually the discussion ends with my mother crying or yelling. My father at least knows to stay calm and collected when he talks to me. If it's not brought up we get along fine and I feel like I'm a normal, productive person. But when being gay comes up, I feel like I'm this freak of nature who has problems. They have this sort of underlying disgust. Their reaction hardens the divide between us."

Aaron's mother keeps hoping he will change and each time he comes home and is "still gay," she is angry and disappointed. Aaron feels her disapproval, shame and disgust. How could he feel good about himself?

If you're experiencing feelings similar to Aaron's mother and don't know where to begin, try saying to your teen, "Look, this is very tough for me, but let's try to talk about what's going on for you." Or you can admit, "I have no idea what this must be like for you, but I'm willing to listen."

To get to the point of being able to listen, you need to find a time and place to work through your feelings of discomfort. Perhaps a counselor, a trusted friend, or parent you met at Parents, Friends and Families of Lesbians and Gays (PFLAG) can be an objective sounding board and support, so you can discuss what's bothering you.

One thing you don't want is a power struggle with your child. No one is going to win that, particularly on something as important as sexual behavior. As soon as you try to control—or even appear to be controlling—your child may withdraw and become isolated from family and even friends. I can't repeat often enough that an isolated child is a child at risk, because he has no one to turn to for support or help. If your child does not withdraw, he may engage in behaviors that you really don't want— just to spite you.

Creating an open atmosphere doesn't guarantee he will talk to you, but there is a greater chance that it will happen, particularly if you show that you are open and accepting of people who are different from you.

Role Model Diversity

When you create an environment that is receptive to people and ideas different from your own, you send a message to your child that he is free to be himself, to be different from you without shame. He will know that he is loved and accepted, even if he follows a path divergent from yours, whether it's his career, his hobbies or his sexual orientation. If he has seen that you respond well to diversity in general, he will be less likely to conclude that he'll be judged badly by you if he is attracted to someone of the same sex.

It is very difficult to "teach" diversity. In fact, you can't teach it unless you live it. Lecturing and giving advice usually backfire. But modeling compassion and tolerance speaks louder than any of your words. Ideally, this process starts when your children are very young and impressionable, but it is not too late to make changes now.

Think about the following areas and try to answer the next series of questions honestly. They may seem trivial but they are indications of the messages you are sending to your family about diversity.

Do you encourage your children to ask questions? Are you annoyed by your children's questions and give as short an answer as possible, or do you see each question as an opportunity for a "teachable moment"? When your child asks a question, the following replies encourage him to be curious:

"I'm so glad you asked."

"That's a great question."

"Let's see. Let me think about that."

You can create an open atmosphere by modeling interactions with a variety of people and by respecting their difference. You want to encourage your children neither to ignore or overemphasize difference. My cousin's child Tommy, age five adores me and my partner. He wanted to take pictures of his family to his school. He was insistent that he have a picture that included Uncle Jeff and Uncle Kevin. Many families would have said, "Oh, I don't know if you want to show that." My cousin found an old picture of us and Tommy went to school and showed off his family. He was proud of his two uncles.

Tommy is learning from an early age that his family isn't something to be ashamed of, nor is it something to overemphasize. He is not saying, "Look at my gay uncle." He is simply presenting the reality of his life to his classmates. And the important thing is, he initiated it. He wanted the picture.

What kinds of experiences do you expose yourself and your family to? Think about how you'd answer the following questions:

What books do you read?

What movies and television shows do you watch?

What foods do you eat?

Are you open to new ideas, new authors, new foods, new restaurants or do you stick with the tried and true?

Are you intellectually curious about things you see, read and experience?

If your answers to these questions lead you to believe that you are not, in fact, open to newness, that conclusion will have implications for you as the parent of a LGBTQ child. It's natural to be stuck in patterns and have specific likes and dislikes, but you are going to have to bend if you are going to be the kind of supportive, understanding parent your child needs.

I am assuming you are reading this book *because* you want to be able to change and because you want to be there for your child. But even people who have the desire to change can experience moments of frustration and discouragement.

Take your time and don't be too harsh on yourself. Think about what holds you back. At the same time begin taking baby steps to broaden your outlook. Try a new ethnic restaurant, see a foreign film, strike up a conversation at work with someone of a different race.

Your job as a parent is to do what's good for your child, whether it is consistent with your motivations and beliefs or not. Your child is not an extension of you, nor is he there to gratify your ego or help you actualize yourself. You are there to help your child become authentic and whole.

But it's not easy to let your child be authentic. All parents have unconscious expectations for their children. Many simply hope their child turns out like them. If you're a doctor, you probably want your son to be a doctor. But maybe he wants to be a massage therapist. That might mean he's not who you wanted him to be or not at all like you—something that can be hard to tolerate even for the most accepting parent.

That, in essence, is the central struggle that a lot of parents, who are straight, face when their child is LGBTQ. It is the struggle to let go and help your child be who he really is. It's challenging to give your blessing to your child when he turns out to be someone you did not envision him to be.

Chapter Two

YOUR TEEN AND
SEXUALITY

A Frank Look at the World of Today's Teen

IN THE TELEVISION SHOW *Dawson's Creek*, it's not uncommon for friendships to shift from platonic to romantic in a
single show. In one episode, pals Karen and Pacey (a guy) go out
on what they call a non-date, which ends with a full-mouth kiss
as they tumble into her apartment and rip each other's clothes
off. In the same episode, Jen has accompanied her good friend
Dawson out of town for a film festival that is showing his documentary. They've checked into an inn for the night—as friends.

After his film wins an award, they discuss why they never hit it
off as a couple. Dawson is sure it's because she was never attracted
to him. Jen can't believe how wrong he is and kisses him to prove
it. In the next scene, they are lying naked in purple silk sheets.

This is prime time television where sexual activity among
young people is a given. Even though it's clear that this group of
friends is in college, teenagers watching this show have got to
think about themselves. If they haven't had sex, they must think
something is wrong with them. If they are sexually active, it reinforces their behavior.

Sexually explicit televisions shows, videos and music are available to teens around the clock. This "new" media is just one piece
of the changing world in which your child lives. In this chapter,

I'll acquaint you with that environment, which may be very different from the one in which you grew up. I'll give you the information you need to understand what your child is dealing with, show you how to educate yourself, and explain why your involvement is critical in helping your child develop into a sexually healthy adult. Last, I'll offer guidelines for talking with your child about sexual issues, including health risks, and setting boundaries.

A NEW WORLD

Some things never change. As young people become aware of their bodies and their sexuality, they experience a natural and healthy urge to explore those feelings. That's been true since Adam and Eve first bit into the apple, and will remain true until the end of time. There's nothing bad or wrong with it. But your child may be grappling with sexual issues that are probably unfamiliar to you. Your child's world is different from what yours was as a teenager in two key ways:

1. The expectations and dialogue around sexuality begin at a much younger age. As we saw with *Dawson's Creek* and as you can also watch on *Felicity* or *Buffy the Vampire Slayer*, young people are portrayed on television as sexual beings, which of course leads teenagers watching the shows to start questioning themselves: "Well, why am I not sexual? Why am I not doing things?" Consequently, students are forced to confront their sexual identity and their sexual behavior in an earlier phase of their life than other generations did.

   In addition, the Clinton-Lewinsky affair brought the subject of oral sex into America's living rooms, forcing parents to confront questions about sexuality from children at younger ages than in the past.

2. Young people have access to much greater knowledge, more information, and have more diverse personal sexual experiences than previous generations. In many cases, they are having sex before they are psychologically ready to deal with the ramifications. They experience tremendous pressure to conform to the mainstream culture and its rigid gender roles. Boys feel compelled to have sex with girls—and boast about it—to demonstrate they're "a real man" (i.e., not gay). Girls latch onto a boyfriend, proof that they couldn't possibly be a lesbian. Questioning teens, pulled in both directions, don't know which feelings to trust or where they belong, so they isolate themselves or hide their anxiety in a new or bizarre (at least, bizarre to you) style of dress.

But do not be fooled by the facade teenagers put up. While it is true that they have more exposure to sexually explicit language and actions at younger and younger ages, there's a big difference between knowing something and understanding it.

Ironically, just as teens are being increasingly bombarded with more information, more and more school systems have withdrawn from their role of educating them: "Abstinence only" curricula, which tell teens little except that they should abstain from sex until marriage, are the norm for education in many states now, thanks to political maneuverings. Teens are increasingly left on their own to figure things out.

WHAT YOU CAN DO

Your task is greater and more important than any V-chip: It is to help your child navigate this new terrain. She needs someone to help her process information and understand the emotional consequences of her actions. If you are not available, she will get her information either from a peer, from a web site, or by herself, struggling through trial and error.

If she must struggle by herself, then she is without the most important part of her support network, you. An alienated child becomes a misinformed child—a child at risk.

NEW FACTS FOR YOU TO DIGEST

In the rest of the chapter, I will give you the information and guidelines to become that educated, informed, involved parent that your child needs and wants. To begin with, here are three factors affecting your child's changing environment.

1. Disconnect Between Physical and Emotional Maturity

One factor that accounts for your child's appearance of sexual precocity is that teenagers are experiencing physiological changes at a younger age. Young women, for example, are going through puberty much earlier than did previous generations. Thus, a well-developed twelve-year-old girl may look as sophisticated as a twenty-year-old, but you have to remember that she's still twelve years old emotionally and treat her as such. In the film *American Beauty,* the young Lolita-like blond cheerleader pretends to have a level of sophistication and sexual experience that she doesn't, in fact, possess. When she is pushed to act as worldly as she looks, her naïveté and fear surface.

As this cheerleader illustrates, just because teens know how to act or have certain information, it doesn't mean they know what to do with it. Ten-year-olds in 2002 are no more prepared to process this information than they were in 1952. They are still ten years old intellectually and emotionally, but they are reacting to a different set of pressures with a different set of information.

Teens feel socially charged to play a particular role at younger ages than they have done before, because they feel they have to prove that they are straight. Their social acceptance is based on proving this. They try to fool their peers, because the social costs—ostracism and isolation—of being LGBTQ are so high. At the same time, they may be fooling themselves. The danger, of course, is that when LGBTQ youth hide their true selves, they must lead a false life, which can lead to serious consequences, including depression.

2. Youth Coming Out Earlier

While there is considerable pressure on teens today to conform to rigid gender roles and prove they're straight, they are also coming out at a younger age. After all, they've grown up with AIDS and Ellen. Whereas once LGBTQ young people struggled in isolation, trying to find a name for their feelings, more and more of them today are highly aware of "what they are" and less willing to hide that. Consequently, they are dealing with their sexual identity and LGBTQ issues much sooner than you probably did.

Studies show that this is not just a theory. The age of first awareness of sexual orientation ranged from 9.6 years to 10.1 years in five university-based studies done during the 1990s. However, because of the pressure to lie and hide that many LGBTQ teens still feel, the age of actually "coming out" (to others) was somewhere between fifteen and seventeen years, which seems to suggest that the age of coming out is heading downward over time.

There's a hidden piece of information in these studies that's important for parents: This statistic means that for five to six years, your child struggled alone with the knowledge that she was LGBTQ. She lived with that secret and she may still be struggling if she hasn't come out to you.

The danger in living with a secret is that it creates a life of lies and deceits. It isolates your child from others. An isolated teen is a teen at risk for problems.

Another new phenomenon has surfaced that you should be aware of. We now have a whole generation of teens who are coming out before they've actually had sex. That is a healthy development, because they are starting to learn that there is a difference between your sexual identity and your sexual behavior: you don't have to have sex to know you're LGBT.

Think about it: You probably knew you were straight years before you had sex. So, it doesn't make sense to ask your child, "How do you know you're gay if you've never had sex?" She knows, just as you know you're straight.

3. New Health Risks

Sexuality over the last twenty years has developed a health aspect that was missing from consciousness when you were a teenager in the 1960s and '70s, thanks to AIDS, hepatitis, and chlamydia, among other diseases. Our knowledge of sexually transmitted diseases (STDs) is much greater, so being sexually active today is much more fraught with risk. I know that raises your anxiety level. But take a deep breath, acknowledge those feelings, and I'll show you how to deal with the reality. Pretending health risks don't exist will not help your child.

Just as young people, for a variety of reasons, are being forced to think about themselves, their sexual identity and their sexual activity at a much younger age, parents are more aware now that there are real dangers attached to sexual behavior. You may be unsettled by the types of questions your child brings home (if she feels comfortable bringing questions home at all—if she does, you're lucky, and have already won half the battle) and concerned because there is real anxiety about what this might mean for your child's life. That is why it is so important to discuss with her the necessity of protecting herself. (I'll explain how to do that in the next section).

WHY YOUR CHILD NEEDS YOU NOW

When LGBTQ teens don't know that their parents care about them, most will find themselves adrift and dangerously vulnerable to the abuse of others in this new environment. In the last chapter, we talked about how to make your home a haven for your child and discussed why that is important for so many reasons.

In the context of your child's sexual behavior, having a safe haven is important for another reason: Youth who feel like they belong and who feel loved are more likely to protect themselves from pregnancy and STDs. Teens who think that no one cares about them or is paying attention to them are careless about protecting their health. This behavior could be a call for attention, an unconscious hope that they'll get sick; only then will they get the attention they need and want from their parents.

I'll never forget talking to one high school junior about the importance of using a condom. He said, "Why should I use a condom? My life isn't worth saving anyway."

You have to think you're a valuable person to say to your partner, whether you are male or female, LGBTQ or straight, "You need to wear a condom because my life is worth living. I want to protect it and control it."

People think that if you just give a young person information about protecting herself, she will take it and run with it. I can't tell you the number of young people who know they are supposed to use a condom and don't.

It is because we are missing the crucial link in educating young people: These are human beings, not machines. They may know they are supposed to use a condom, but they still have to make a choice to do so.

It is not just a question of telling your child how to use a condom or why using a condom is important. It is a question of helping your child believe that her life matters enough to put that knowledge to actual use. As a parent, you can do this in several ways:

- If your child is in a play at school or is receiving an award, arrange your schedule so you can be in the audience, even if it means missing a couple of hours of work.
- Go to the open house at your child's school. Sit in her seat, meet her teachers and come back with comments for your child.
- Give meaningful praise, based on "camera check feedback" (feedback so clear that someone could take a picture of the event you're describing and see it) about things you see your child is doing. Make statements like, "I was really proud of how you handled the pressure around preparing for the exam" or "You did a great job of cleaning up the kitchen after your party." These kinds of specific comments mean a lot more than a generic "You're a great kid."
- Don't belittle her feelings or her world: Things that may not seem like a big deal to you are a big deal to her and, if you say they aren't, it makes the young person feel devalued.
- Tell your child you love her every day.

BASIC INFORMATION YOU NEED

In order to comprehend the sexual identity issues your child is struggling with, you need to have some basic information. The following two key concepts about sexuality will give you a foundation and a perspective for understanding her experiences and struggles. Key concepts about gender identity will be discussed in Chapter 6.

1. A Healthy Sexual Identity

Sexuality has three basic parts:

    a. sexual orientation (the attraction one feels toward either or both sexes)
    b. sexual behavior (the sex acts one engages in, alone or with others)
    c. sexual identity (how one sees oneself and how others recognize one).

In healthy development, sexual orientation, behavior and identity are all in harmony. But many LGBTQ youth experience a disconnect between their orientation and their behavior and identity, forcing them to hide their secret. This isolates them and puts them at higher risk for problems.

No reputable scientific or psychiatric authority today thinks that sexual orientation changes or that your sexual orientation is a choice, although this is a common misconception. What happens is that people come to terms with their sexual orientation and make decisions about behavior and identity at different phases over the course of a lifetime. That means that people may deal with it at different times in their lives, and may choose to communicate that information in different ways at those times, as Tim illustrates in the following story.

Tim, thirty-seven, denied that he was gay throughout high school and college, although he did have sex with a few guys there. He was married for seven years; everyone thought he was straight. "I married to keep my family happy," he says. "I had known for years on some level that I was gay, but for me to accept it and finally go, 'This is what I am'—I just couldn't do it. I definitely tried to shove that feeling deep, deep inside because of what society thought. As a kid growing up in a church-oriented, God-fearing family, I always heard, 'Being gay is wrong, wrong, wrong.' "

Now Tim realizes he was hiding behind the guise of being straight. He came out following his divorce five years ago, and is now living with a man. For the first time in his life, he feels at peace. Tim's orientation never changed; his behavior and identity did. He made a choice to hide his sexual identity.

Your child, too, may know that she is LGBTQ but may choose not to act on it or announce it to you. That is where the element of choice comes in around behavior. Because of the pressure to appear straight in high school, many LGBTQ youth remain closeted. Their orientation is homosexual but their behavior may make them appear straight: they may date someone of the opposite sex and others may see them as straight (their identity). It can be very detrimental and confusing to act one way and know inside that this is not who you truly are.

2. The Sexuality Continuum

Sexuality is not black or white. There is much more fluidity than people generally recognize. When Alfred Kinsey and his associates did their groundbreaking work on sexuality in the late 1940s and the early 1950s, they found that no one is purely straight or purely gay, that most of us have attractions contrary to our primary sexual orientation and many have sexual experiences with the same or both sexes. More recent research by Masters and Johnson and others have supported Kinsey's results. He developed a six-point continuum based on the degree of sexual responsiveness people have to members of their own sex and to the opposite sex.

If you consider yourself exclusively heterosexual you would be at the far left, 0, and if you are exclusively homosexual, you would rate a 6. If you are mainly heterosexual but have a few homosexual experiences, you would probably be a 1 or 2 depending on the duration and extent of those experiences. The same is true on the other end: If you are gay and also have straight experiences occasionally, you might fall into 4 or 5. Bisexuals land somewhere in the middle range.

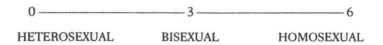

0 ——————————————— 3 ——————————————— 6

HETEROSEXUAL   BISEXUAL   HOMOSEXUAL

Keep this continuum in mind as you read this book and as you meet others who will try to fit your child into a rigid sexuality box. The reality is that there is not a neatly drawn line between gay and straight and everyone falls on one side or the other. There are people who do and are also people who fall all along the continuum. For example, you can be emotionally attracted to members of the same sex without wanting to have sex with them.

HOW YOU CAN EDUCATE YOURSELF

There are two parts to educating yourself: understanding the sexual continuum and informing yourself about your child's culture. Both are equally important.

You don't have to remain hopelessly in the dark ages. At the same time, you don't want to start acting or dressing like a sixteen-year-old. That will not endear you to your teenager. The following guidelines will help you to better understand your child's world and give you the tools to cope with what you are learning. They will also give you the information and confidence to talk with your child about sexual issues and behavior, which will be covered later in this chapter.

Spend time understanding the culture your child lives in. Here are four ways to begin this process:

1. Watch some episodes of the television shows teens watch, such as *Temptation Island, Buffy the Vampire Slayer* or *Dawson's Creek.*

2. Listen to her music with an open mind.

3. Go to the web sites she frequents.

4. Find a chat room on AOL and listen in. Planetout.
   com is a favorite web site among LGBTQ teens.

Do this on your own time. I don't recommend you watch television shows with her. There is a big difference between understanding what your child is seeing and talking about it, and appearing to condone it. Watching a show with your child could cause her to withdraw and could also could give the appearance that you approve of what she's watching.

I'm also not suggesting, however, you say, "I want to watch that before you watch it." Nothing makes a teenager want to watch something more than having it declared "off limits" by her parents, so your attempts to censor what she sees or reads probably will only backfire. But on your own time, watch it just to see what images concern you. If you tell her, "I don't want you watching that show," that is probably not going to be terribly effective anyhow. She'll just watch it at a friend's house.

It's better to see the show yourself, understand it, and try to figure out the extent to which your child might be troubled, confused or titillated by what she sees, and then talk about it with her. You can open the discussion by saying something like, "I was surfing channels the other night and happened to see part of (insert TV show). I was troubled by . . . Do you ever watch that? What do you think?" See what she says.

If you are disturbed by what you see, however, don't necessarily assume that your child is. I remember once watching *South Park* with my high-school-age nephew. I froze when a particular innuendo was used, but then I realized it had passed over his head because he didn't even know the term. Sometimes teens laugh just because their friends are laughing; they don't even know what they're laughing at. If you're watching a television show or video together and see or hear something that disturbs you, follow these three steps:

1. Observe your child's reaction: Did she react at all? Is she laughing? Does she seem upset?

2. Note it. If she does not react, she may have missed the point, like my nephew, so you can let it pass. If she seems upset, you can simply say, "That scene about . . . seemed to upset you" and let her respond. If she's laughing and you're not sure she gets it, you can ask her: "What's so funny? I don't get it," and see if she can explain it to you.

3. Depending on her reaction, talk to her about what she is seeing and what she understands.

Understand the language your child uses. Many terms have very different meanings today than when you were growing up. Remember "Getting to first base"? The quaint language of yesteryear—getting to first base is kissing, second base is sexual touching above the waist and third base is sexual touching below the waist—has gone the way of the dinosaur and the Edsel.

The significance of oral sex has changed drastically in the last fifteen years. Did you know that the term "hooking up" means oral sex to a lot of teens? And that oral sex is not considered sex by more than half of college undergrads, according to one study? According to another survey of college freshmen and sophomores in the South, more than a third think of oral sex as abstinence.

As a result of not perceiving oral sex as intimate, youth don't recognize the health risks and don't protect themselves.

To learn the new language of your teen, do the following:

1. Listen closely during the carpool or at other times when teens may talk in uninhibited ways, then ask questions of your child later, to understand what they were saying. You can bring it up casually later. While you're making dinner, you can say, "Gee, that was an interesting com-

ment Stacey made in the car today. What do you think she meant when she said . . . ? "

2. Familiarize yourself with the places teens get their information, such as TV shows, movies, the Internet, and publications like *YM* magazine.

3. Talk to other parents to see what they know.

Find out what kind of sex education your child is getting at school. There is great variety in sex ed courses among high schools. Most schools do a frightfully bad job in this area, which means the burden falls back to you. Some schools teach "abstinence only" education. There is no evidence that "abstinence only" education reduces the likelihood of teen pregnancy or STDs, but may instead deny young people life-saving information.

If you are not embarrassed or uncomfortable (many parents are, but still go in), I urge you to go into school and talk with the principal and teacher. Ask to see the syllabus, and determine whether you feel the course is preparing your child for the real world. If it is not, follow the steps in Chapter 9 about how to initiate a change at your child's school.

Remember that sex education does not lead to more sexual activity, just safer and healthier interactions.

HOW TO TALK WITH YOUR CHILD ABOUT SEXUAL ISSUES

Most parents want their children to have information about sex, sexuality and relationships but are often uncomfortable discussing these topics. Recent research from the Kaiser Family Foundation showed that most teens wanted more information about sex from their parents and that parents were starting much too late and not talking nearly enough. You may not know where to begin the discussion if you didn't start it when your child was younger.

But there's a very good reason to do it now: Studies show that teens who feel they can talk with their parents about sex are less likely to engage in high-risk behavior than teens who feel they can't talk with their parents about the subject.

Here is a list of five Dos and Don'ts to help you open a dialogue about this very sensitive topic:

DON'T think you need to sit down and have The Big Talk.
DO look for "teachable moments" and make the most of them.

Sitting your child down and saying, "We need to talk about sex" is sure to make you nervous and her clam up. Instead, look for instances in your everyday life—television shows, articles in the newspaper, incidents at school—that relate to sex, sexuality or sexual health. Keep your ears open and use these instances as a way to open the discussion. For example, if two girls are discussing whether to sleep with their boyfriends on one of the teen television shows, you might make a comment like, "Isn't it interesting that they haven't discussed ways to protect themselves?" See what your teen says in response. At some point in your discussion, you can say, "Whether you're LGBTQ or straight, you need to protect yourself."

DON'T act like you have all the information.
DO admit you're uncomfortable discussing this.

If you can't overcome your discomfort—and this is a subject that is difficult for many parents to discuss—admit it to your child. It will make you seem human, and your honesty may allow her also to admit that she's uncomfortable talking about it with you too. It's okay to say something like, "You know, I'm uncomfortable talking about sex because my parents never talked with me about it. But I want us to be able to talk about anything—including sex—so please, come to me if you have any questions. And if I don't know the answer, I'll find out or we can find out together."

If you don't know the answer to one of her questions, admit it. Just say, "That's a new one for me. I honestly don't know. Let's find out together [or] I'll look it up and let you know."

DON'T dryly recite factual information.
DO communicate your values.

Research shows that children want and need moral guidance from their parents, so don't hesitate to make your beliefs and values clear. For example, you can communicate the psychological and emotional repercussions of having intercourse for the wrong reasons by saying:

To your daughter: "Girls who have intercourse early often feel exploited and used as though they've lost control of their bodies."

To a son or daughter: "If you have intercourse to please your partner or because you think he'll like you more if you do, that doesn't always work, and you might end up regretting that decision. You should do things because you want to do them, not because someone else wants you to."

To a son or daughter: "Some kids think they can trade sex for popularity or status, but that usually backfires. It often just brings you a lot of pain and disappointment."

After you've made your point, follow these four steps:

1. Observe her reaction.

2. Note it by saying something like, "You seem upset by my comment" or "You seem surprised by what I said."

3. Ask her if that has happened to anyone she knows.

4. Share an incident from your youth about what happened to you or a friend in a similar situation.

If your child is open enough to tell you that she believes that oral sex is harmless, or that she can do it and still be a virgin so it's not a big deal, you can gently bring in its seriousness and help her to think about the emotional consequences by saying something like, "There are many steps in sexual activity. It's true that oral sex isn't intercourse but it is still powerful and emotional and can affect your relationship."

Some teens may describe "friends" who engage in certain activities to test your reaction. Don't assume that these are real "friends" (she might be speaking about herself), or that she even knows anyone actually engaging in these behaviors. Just take the comment at face value and respond by giving advice as described above.

DON'T give erroneous messages to scare your child.
DO give her the truth.

It's been proven over and over again that scare tactics about public health education—such as, if you have homosexual sex you'll automatically get AIDS or if you smoke pot once you'll become a heroin addict—are ineffective in the long run, because when young people finally do cross that boundary, they find out the warning is usually exaggerated or not true at all. As a result, they lose faith completely in the authority figure who gave them the erroneous message. Your credibility as a parent is important: You must give an accurate message, which is not extreme and not meant to cause panic but to inform.

DON'T sanitize your youth.
DO keep appropriate boundaries but share some of your youthful struggles.

A lot of parents make a big mistake by pretending that their childhood was more innocent than it was. All that really does is lead your child to believe that you're hopelessly out of it and could never understand her world or be of any help.

You must walk a fine line. You want to maintain some boundaries and not go into every little thing you did when you were younger. (You will have to use your own judgment here in terms of defining an appropriate boundary.) But in a suitable and restrained way, let your child know that you grappled with a lot of the same issues when you were her age, even though you may have done things in a more innocent form. This lets your child know you're a real human being who makes mistakes too.

The more you present the world that you grew up in as somehow totally different from the world she is growing up in, the less likely she is to listen to you as someone who has anything to offer in terms of guidance.

Some parents think that if they don't reveal their own vulnerabilities, weaknesses or mistakes when they were younger, that their child will somehow respect them more. That's just not true.

If you say, "I can't believe this, we would never have done this at your age," first of all, you're probably lying, and second, you're playing into her natural wish to differentiate herself from you. A key task of adolescence is to establish an identity independent of parents and family, and responses like this one may simply lead her to go ahead and do it anyway, as a way of separating from you.

Instead, I recommend you say, "Look, I don't necessarily have all the answers, but I have faced many of the same questions when I was your age, and people have faced these questions throughout eternity, and everybody has to grapple with them." You can go on and say, "I had a really hard time with them and here are some of my experiences." Then describe some of your experiences.

You can also add, "I would probably do some things differently now if I had to do them over again, but I didn't know then what I know now. You'll probably make some decisions that you'll regret, too." Then you can talk about the consequences of unsafe sex, for example. You might also add that some of these consequences are much sterner than when you were young. Without scaring her, you want to recognize that there is an element of danger today that you didn't have to face.

DISCUSSING HEALTH RISKS

Many studies have found that an individual's episodes of unsafe sex correspond to his or her feelings of social isolation and low self-esteem.* Since many LGBTQ teens feel socially isolated and suffer from low self-esteem, they are particularly at risk for engaging in unsafe sexual behavior.

If you're the parent of a daughter, that may surprise you. The facts are: LGBTQ adolescent women are at twice as high a risk for unwanted pregnancy than straight teens (12 percent vs. 5.3 percent). They also have a higher incidence of physical abuse (19 percent vs. 12 percent) and sexual abuse (22 percent vs. 13 percent) than straight teens.†

You may wonder why a young woman who knows she's not straight is having sex with boys. Mary, a seventeen-year-old high school senior explains why she did it: "I've known I'm a lesbian, probably all of my life. But I've had boyfriends, too. In fact, I did have sex with one of them, at the age of fourteen. I've now come to realize I only did it because I was confused. The thing is, I didn't like it. I've had sex a number of times since then. I never liked it. So why did I do it? Because I thought I *should* like it. I wanted to be normal, and like it. But I didn't."

Many lesbian and bisexual teens may have sex because they feel they should or because they're trying to "cure" themselves of their homosexual attractions. Others have heterosexual intercourse because they don't yet identify themselves as a lesbian or bisexual. Some are forced to have sex.

That means that no matter what her orientation, your daughter needs to protect herself from unwanted pregnancy, sexually transmitted diseases and abuse.

And so does your son. According to one study, sexually trans-

---

* Lipkin, Arthur, p. 159.
† Information from *The Washington Blade*, 7/2/99.

mitted diseases infect almost 50 percent of gay and bisexual teens between the ages of fifteen and nineteen.*

I'm giving you this statistic, in part, to scare you. I want you to realize the necessity of talking with your teen about safe sex.

This is not an easy discussion to have. It's hard for straight parents to talk to straight kids about sex because it's such a private topic. It's even harder for straight parents and LGBTQ teens to talk because they don't have a shared experience.

But it is a very necessary discussion. Here are the five steps to take:

1. Inform yourself first. Make sure that you have the latest information on STDs, HIV infection, pregnancy prevention and AIDS. Check the back of the book for resources, web sites and hotlines that can give you the information you need.

2. Begin by saying something like, "Do you have a few minutes? There's something I'd like to talk to you about." Then you can say, "I've been reading about the high rate of STDs/HIV infection/pregnancy/in teenage boys/girls and I want to be sure you have the facts and know how to protect yourself." See where she takes it from here.

3. Remember to frame the discussion in a health context, not a moral one. Try to avoid judging comments, such as "You should . . ." or "You what?" or "How could you?" Please go back to Chapter 1 and read the section on how to keep your own values out of the discussion if this is an issue for you.

4. If you're feeling uncomfortable with the topic, admit your discomfort. Say something like, "This is really hard for me, but I feel it's a discussion we need to have."

5. Leave the door open for further discussions. When you

* Lipkin, Arthur, p. 158.

sense that you are near the end of the conversation or that your teen is getting restless, say, "Let's table this for now and talk again later" or "We've covered enough for today. Let's talk again in a few days."

Keep the following points in mind as well:

• No matter how your teen reacts to the discussion—whether you were rebuffed or greeted with an icy stare—remember that she heard you. Give yourself credit for opening the door to a sensitive, difficult subject. It will get easier next time.

• If your teen won't talk to you, make sure that she has *someone* to talk to. Issues of sexuality are notoriously difficult for teens to discuss with their parents; an older sibling, peer educator, trusted relative or similar person can be an important resource.

Your job is to make sure she has access to that resource—you don't always have to be that resource yourself. You can say to her, "I know this is a hard discussion for us. You're really close to Aunt Sally, maybe you can talk to her better. If you make plans to see her, I'll drive you over to her house."

YOU DID FINE

No matter how your discussions are faring, you will probably feel that you could have done better. That's a natural reaction. Since the dawn of time parents have felt they've screwed up with their children, yet somehow both parents and children have survived. No one is the perfect parent. No one is ever going to do all of this right. This is a very difficult subject for both parents and children to discuss with each other.

Your child wants to see that you are trying. She understands that you're going to make mistakes. She's seen you make plenty already. So, cut yourself some slack. There will always be another time to initiate a discussion if you didn't pick up on something when you thought you should have. You can always go back to your child and say, "You know, I was thinking about something I said the other night . . ." and admit you goofed. The important thing is that you care enough about your child and her sexual development to open up a dialogue, share your values and experiences, and listen to her.

SET BOUNDARIES

Throughout all of the dialogues and activities I have suggested in this chapter runs a constant thread: the need for a sense of boundaries. All children need to know that a solid set of rules and standards governs their home. They want to know what they can do and what they cannot do. When they don't have structure, they panic. They may rebel against structure but deep down, they want it because otherwise it feels like things are out of control and nobody is in charge.

Especially for teens, boundaries give them stability when so much of their life is in flux. It shows them that you care enough to say "No." When teens and pre-teens don't know what the boundaries are or when they seem to be enforced in an arbitrary and capricious manner, they feel as though they've lost their rudder.

I cannot tell you what your particular boundaries should be. You will need to work that out based on your values, your family and your culture.

Here are guidelines for responding to a boundary that has been crossed. Say that you received an enormous credit card bill one month and learned that your sixteen-year-old son had been logging onto pornographic sites and charging them to your card.

1. Calmly repeat the rule that has been broken: "There are two issues here: You have used my credit card without my permission and I am concerned that you are viewing porn. You know you are not allowed to use my credit card without asking me first. We've also talked about your not surfing pornographic sites. You have broken both of these rules."

2. Explain your reasons for having them by continuing, "The credit card belongs to me and is for my use only. If you want to use it for something, you need to ask my permission. It is not a good idea for you to access pornographic sites at your age. That material is for older adults."

3. Then, state the consequences: "As a result of breaking these rules you will lose your driving privileges for two weeks" or "You are grounded for the next two weekends."

If your child is the type who tries to persuade you to change your mind about the consequences, try not to get into a discussion with her. State the rules and if you need to, leave the room.

Keep in mind that teenagers are going to cross boundaries. There's nothing you can do about it—other than be prepared to handle the situation when it arises.

Chapter Three

YOUR TEEN AND SOCIETY

How Cultural Messages about Gender
and Sexuality Affect Your Teen

A S A C H I L D, I was very athletic and loved sports. On my eighth birthday, I wanted to go to the YMCA with my dad to play sports all day. We played basketball together. Then my father went into the swimming pool to cool off. He had a heart attack in the pool and died on my eighth birthday.

I was understandably devastated, baffled and overwhelmed and didn't know how to behave.

At the funeral, I started to cry. My older brother, who was twenty, turned to me and said, "Don't cry. Be a man. Don't be a faggot."

I may have had a little bit of an inkling I was gay. I was already given a very clear message of how you were supposed to act if you were a young man. That included not crying at your father's funeral when you're eight.

I don't remember crying in front of anybody again for ten years. I didn't want anyone to think that I was a faggot. I wanted everyone to think I was a real man. In my brother's defense, I must say that he was probably doing what my father told him to do: He was trying to teach his little brother how to behave if you're a male in our society.

Long before I had any real understanding of issues of sexual orientation, I was beginning to see how cultural expectations around gender and appropriate behavior for girls and boys get mixed in with issues of sexual orientation. In this chapter, we'll examine how these myths and gender stereotypes, including some of the subtle assumptions, can influence your child rearing. This information and the awareness you gained in the first chapter can help you free your child so he is not squeezed into a gender or orientation box that is inappropriate, uncomfortable, or downright damaging to him.

STRAIGHT UNTIL PROVEN OTHERWISE

Heterosexism, the assumptions that everyone is heterosexual and conforms to traditional gender roles, is so omnipresent that it is "invisible." For example, on the Long Island Railroad I saw an ad for frozen dinners. It read, "Remember when you generously said you'd share the cooking? No? Well, she sure does." It seems innocent enough, but on closer look, you see that it's based on the assumption that everyone on the train is straight, married and that they relate in a certain way: that men don't cook and women do the household chores. Anyone who's LGBTQ on that train and understands the ad will feel alienated (I'm sure that many heterosexuals, especially women, are offended as well).

The disturbing thing about heterosexism is that it is invisible to the people who have the privilege. When married couples walk hand in hand, we don't consider them making a political statement. Yet if two gay men walk down the street holding hands, people say, "Why do they have to flaunt it?" Heterosexism is one of a series of "unearned privileges" that individuals in our society receive simply because they were born into groups that are privileged.

Our culture defines gender in large part in reference to sexual identity and sexual behavior. We cannot separate our ideas of "real men" and "real women" from our beliefs about sexual orientation and behavior. For many people, what makes you a man is that you're not gay. What makes you a real woman is that you're not a lesbian. Thus, caring, sensitive behavior in men is equated with being gay, and aggressive, assertive behavior in women is conflated with being a lesbian. These stereotypes become a way of straitjacketing people of both genders and all sexual orientations, because obviously all women have an assertive side and all men have a sensitive side.

These ingrained cultural notions are amplified in teens, who need their peers' approval to validate their own shaky sense of self. These unchallenged and unspoken assumptions may underlay your parenting as well. Have you ever said to your school-age son, "Do you have a girlfriend?" or "Which girl do you think is cute?" Such questions send an unspoken expectation that you assume your child is straight.

GENDER STEREOTYPES

Gender stereotypes set expectations for behavior. Because these stereotypes are so pervasive and so constant, parents can perpetuate them without even realizing it.

You cannot control television shows, videos or magazine ads and articles. But you have the power to challenge the narrow views presented by the mass media and other institutions, which can eat away at a child's self-esteem and self-confidence. Counteract the negative messages your child is hearing with positive ones.

What you say matters to your teen. He may brush you off or laugh at your comment, but be sure: He's heard you. Your child's friends do have an influence on him, but so do you. Teenagers want to know where their parents stand on important issues.

Use your influence to recognize stereotypic behavior and encourage your child to be authentic.

Here are some of the most conspicuous stereotypes and what you can do to combat them:

School Performance

For many years, both parents and teachers ushered boys into math and science courses and steered girls into the "softer" classes, such as art and writing. Math was thought too difficult for girls, and the arts were considered for "sissies." If a boy took an art course, he was considered gay ("a sissy"), the worst thing a boy could be in the eyes of his straight peers.

These stereotypes force your child into a gender straitjacket that prevents him from expressing who he really is and may lead him to live a double life. Not all eighth-grade girls are boy crazy, for example, and not all tenth-grade boys just want a piece of the action. They may just act that way to be accepted by their peers.

Magazines

Magazine covers are interchangeable. The women's

> **TIP:** Encourage your daughter to follow her natural inclination and your son to take the courses that excite him. One way to do this is to ask your child what courses his friends are taking. Then say, "Do you want to take what your friends are taking?" Or, "Have you thought about taking something different from what your friends are taking?"
>
> See if he is following his friends because he is generally interested in the course, or because he feels social pressure when all the girls or all the boys are taking certain courses.
>
> If it's the latter, encourage him to do what feels right to him, rather than what someone else thinks he should do. Say something like, "There will be many times in your life when you'll have to choose between doing what's popular and what everyone else is doing, and what you really want to do in your heart. I know it's difficult to be different from your friends, but if you follow your heart, you will never go wrong." You might also give him an example from your life of when you did something against peer pressure and how you benefited.

gleam with beautiful, slim, white women with perfect teeth and nary a blemish. The men's magazines sport handsome hunks with glistening muscular bodies on their covers. In all fairness, it must be said that occasionally some of these magazines do tackle issues of substance. *Seventeen* offered resources for girls coming out as lesbians. *Teen* ran an article on how to fight for your legal and criminal rights in school. Unfortunately, this type of article is still the exception to pages that are ruled by advice on makeup and wardrobe selection.

The ads continue to push products in a gender-specific way. In an interesting case study of Clinique toiletry products, two British researchers noted how the cosmetic company "coded" advertisements for male and female products differently so they would conform to what is acceptable behavior for men and women.

The ads for male products carried more information about the product, presenting new aspects as factual reporting. They stressed the usefulness and efficiency of the product, often using the language of business, such as in suggesting "an important meeting" with a bar of soap. The male ads used more rough and tough images, with names like, "Face Scrub" or "Scruffing Lotion."

Women's products, in contrast, suggested soft and sensual and played on the notions of purity and cleanliness with such names as "Cream Cleanser." Their ads used fewer words and conveyed the message with only

> **TIP:** If you see your children reading a popular magazine, remind them that these are models, that real boys are not that muscular and that most girls are not that thin. Ask them to contrast what they see on the pages of magazines with what they see in the real world around them, and help them understand that these idealized images are just that—idealized.
>
> Encourage them to develop other aspects of their personalities besides concentrating on their looks. This is a good way to engage yourself in your child's life in a way that is comforting and active without being confrontational or critical.

a photo of the product.* They reinforce stereotypical notions about women: that they are soft and cuddly and make emotional decisions. But perhaps, more important, the lack of written information shows that women don't need facts about a product, because they've been indoctrinated into the need for makeup, toners and moisturizers from a young age by reading the women's magazines and listening to their older sisters or mothers talk.

GREAT EXPECTATIONS

Kelli, who came out as a lesbian in college, learned what most children realize by the time they become teenagers: gender identity is equated with sexual identity. A young woman shows that she's a real woman by acting feminine. A key component of that is active heterosexual behavior and identity: having sex with guys and making sure everyone knows what she's doing.

Kelli's story may help you understand what your daughter is going through. She explains how expectations about female appearance affected her. "I feared I was gay in high school, so I always made sure I had lipstick on. I didn't like wearing makeup, but I didn't want to be perceived as a dyke."

Kelli got the message loud and clear: lipstick/femininity, sexy to men. No lipstick/dyke.

In elementary school, she was a tomboy. "My parents indulged that: I had matchbox cars, all my friends were boys. I wore cord pants and Izod shirts," she remembers. "But when I started to get breasts—I had long hair at twelve or thirteen—my mom started pushing me: 'Oh, you're so pretty, why don't you wear this skirt or that dress.' I didn't like wearing skirts, but at the

* Kirkham, Pat and Alex Weller, "Cosmetics: A Clinique Case Study" in *The Gendered Object*, pp. 196–203.

same time, I was pleasing everyone else, so I felt good. I *did* look good in dresses. But I knew deep down that wasn't who I was."

In the seventh grade, Kelli realized she was out of sync with the other girls in her class: She noticed that all her friends were boys. She said to herself, this is not normal. I'm supposed to be dating boys and talking about them with my girlfriends. She made a conscious effort to make friends with girls, and from then on, had a social circle of girlfriends.

Kelli's behavior is typical of a girl who suspects she might be a lesbian. But like most teens, she wants to be accepted and liked by her peers and have her parents' approval and so she denies and hides her true feelings. Kelli did all the things her straight girl friends did, just to prove she wasn't a lesbian. No one had to tell her what to do: she simply conformed to acceptable female behavior in this society.

Her mother also pushed her to comply—not because she's a bad mom, but because she herself had been taught from an early age that traditional gender behavior was the key to happiness for young women. Her mother may also not realize that young people today have more freedom to "bend" gender roles because they are less defined than when parents were their age.

For a guy, proving his masculinity means showing that he's not gay. Dan played that part well. His story may shed light on your son's. He grew up on a military base with a macho dad who loved football. Dan wasn't interested in sports. He preferred to stay at home and cook with his mom. Fortunately, his sister was a sports fanatic and served as a companion to their dad. But still, Dan says, "I was taught that men should be tough and masculine and kind of stoic and not show a lot of emotions. I learned to tuck my emotions away."

From the age of twelve on, Dan and his best friend, Ted, had sex two to three times a week in the bushes behind Dan's house. No one knew. Dan played the charade of being straight all through middle and high school. He explains, "I played tennis, I wrestled, and I was on student council. I would date girls for the prom, but I never had a steady girlfriend. I'd asked the same girls out to two or three dances throughout the year, but there was never anything intense about it. I would take her out to dinner, open the door, pay for dinner, take her home and do all that stuff. I followed the basic rules, even though I was doing all this other stuff on the side. I never told anyone about it. The only other person who knew about it was Ted."

No one at school suspected that he might be gay. He says, "I never hit on any boys or gave any indication I was attracted, other than just being buddies or friends. I was never picked on. I was always a big kid too. I'm about six foot five and in high school I was overweight. Being involved in sports and being a letterman and having all that typical macho crap, I just didn't get picked on very much at all."

Despite "passing" as straight, Dan was living behind a suit of armor that hid who he really was. He lived a life of lies and deceits, a primary cause of debilitating depression in teens.

Kelli and Dan worked hard to hide their sexual orientation for one simple reason: they were well aware of the prejudice against people who are LGBT. Beginning as young as kindergarten kids tell each other, "Oh, that's so gay" without understanding what the words mean. They know enough, however, to realize that the phrase is negative and hurtful, and will probably pass without a reprimand.

A LOOK AT THE HISTORY OF ANTI-LGBT BIAS

You, too, are probably well aware of the anti-LGBT bias that pervades our culture and fearful that your child may be hurt because he is LGBTQ. Part of you may even wish your child would "cover up" his sexual preference, just to make everything easier. That's a natural desire but does not help your child.

Meaning well, some parents—often unconsciously—put their children in gender straitjackets to protect them from discrimination and pain. But, of course, the straitjacket is even more damaging to children, because it asks them to learn to do what they are supposed to do, rather than what they're actually good at. They act, dress and walk in ways that are uncomfortable for them—just so others will like them. They internalize the message that the person they know themselves to be is not acceptable. Naturally, from there, self-esteem plummets and sadness, anger and depression take over.

It's important that you know the history of anti-LGBT bias in this country, so you have a context for understanding what your child must endure every day at school. (If your child experiences violence, remember that 80 percent of all LGBT teens experience physical, verbal or sexual harassment while at school, according to the GLSEN 2001 School Climate Survey.) I believe that anti-LGBT bias is based on stereotypes of LGBTQ people, myths about the causes of homosexuality and a lack of personal contact with LGBTQ people.

Men and women have been attracted to the same sex throughout history and their behaviors were either tolerated or prohibited, but they, themselves, were not identified as having a different, separate identity because of their sexual behavior. When you hear the names of Alexander the Great, Michelangelo, and Virginia Woolf, your first thought is not that that person was a homosexual but of their achievement and place in history.

In fact, while there have been people who have had same sex desires and acted on them throughout recorded history, the word homosexual did not exist prior to the nineteenth century. It has only been in the past 150 years, with the growth of industrialism, that people have the means to live outside of traditional nuclear families and have developed what we call the "gay lifestyle." It includes being open about same-sex orientation and talking about it, and living outside of heterosexual marriage, often in a same-sex relationship.

As the "gay lifestyle" spread, LGBTQ people gravitated to each other and set up their own social networks. These communities gave them support, but it also identified them as a minority subculture and thus, made them a target of the larger culture's prejudices.*

In the first half of the twentieth century, people who were LGBTQ were thought to be mentally ill. Attempts at cures and treatments included involuntary imprisonment, drugs and shock therapies. By mid–twentieth century, political leaders saw homosexual behavior as subversive. Senator Joseph McCarthy and his homosexual assistant, Roy Cohn, searched for and outed homosexuals in government service. Some lost their jobs; others committed suicide. With state-sponsored persecution, homophobia became an "acceptable prejudice." By the 1960s, 82 percent of American men and 58 percent of women believed that only Communists and atheists were more dangerous than homosexuals.† This is the very reason that parents don't want their sons and daughters to be LGBTQ—they fear they will be endangered.

Novels and plays portrayed LGBTQ people as perverts, criminals or lunatics whose lives usually ended in either murder or suicide. In response to increasing violence against homosexuals, the gay liberation movement developed. The first American gay rights group was founded in Chicago in 1924, a sort of preview of "coming attractions" as LGBTQ people organized and increasingly fought for equality as the century wore on. A strong community and subculture developed, inspiring a conservative backlash that is still strong today—another fear for parents.

Yet despite this opposition, the public's dislike for LGBTQ people has declined while its support for equality has grown over the past three decades.‡ A few numbers bear this out: Throughout the 1970s and 1980s, disapproval rates were consistently

* Hardin, Kimeron N., Ph.D., p. 47.
† Fone, Byrne, (intro).
‡ Yang, Alan S., p. i.

high, peaking at 75 percent in the late 1980s. A 2001 Gallup poll shows movement toward more tolerance: 85 percent of Americans support equal opportunity in the workplace, 54 percent say homosexual relations between consenting adults should be legal and 52 percent say homosexuality is an acceptable "alternative lifestyle."* Yet in a national survey of 1000 parents by Lake, Shell and Perry, a public opinion polling firm in Washington, D.C., only 26 percent said they would be accepting if their child told them he was gay.†

Why is homosexuality disturbing to so many Americans? The reasons are complex. People often distrust someone who is different; consider the prejudice against blacks, Jews and women. Homosexuality also challenges traditional gender roles and the heterosexism discussed earlier. Traditional families, in which the man and woman take on conventional male and female roles, can feel threatened when two men or two women pair up.

In addition, sex is a highly charged topic in America under any circumstances. Generally speaking, more taboos, fears and repressions exist in this area than any others,‡ so people react with more visceral emotions where sex is concerned. For some, homophobia may mask their discomfort with their own sexual impulses. But because this is too threatening to acknowledge, they project their fears onto LGBTQ people, calling them "sick" or "perverted," or they hide under the guise of religious rhetoric and call them sinful.

MYTHS ABOUT BEING GAY OR LESBIAN

As a parent of an LGBTQ child, it is important that you know the myths surrounding homosexuality and its causes, so you

---

* Info from press release, June 4, 2001.
† National Survey, Horizons Foundation, p. 19.
‡ Bernstein, p. 20.

don't unknowingly perpetuate them. Most of us have grown up influenced by the prejudices of our families, religion and culture, or with biases of our own. At one time, you may have laughed at an anti-gay joke without a second thought or saw AIDS as only a LGBT issue.

In the following section, I will present the most common myths about homosexuality, bisexuality and questioning youth followed by the facts, and tips for handling issues related to the myths should they arise in your family. Please see Chapter 6 for misconceptions about transgendered people.

MYTH: People choose to be gay or lesbian.

FACT: No reputable scientific or psychiatric authority, from the American Psychological Association (APA) on down, thinks people make a choice about their sexual orientation. Orientation is innate and fixed. But people do come to terms with their sexual orientation and make decisions around behavior and identity over the course of a lifetime.

> **TIP:** Teenagers do choose whom they tell and how they act on the knowledge that they're gay or lesbian. A child may know he's gay or lesbian deep down, but may not tell you, because he feels the news will not be accepted. He may secretly have a boyfriend or hide his orientation by dating girls. The best thing you can do is to try to create an open atmosphere at home. See Chapter 1 for details.

MYTH: Homosexuality is caused by a neurotic family background or some other family failing.

FACT: Family background has little or no effect on a person's sexual orientation.* The idea that homosexuality is a

---

* Griffin et al., p. 24.

parent's fault originated in psychoanalytic studies done in the 1960s that found that an engulfing mother and a weak or distant father created a gay or lesbian child. This theory has been discarded as we learn more about sexual orientation.

It has been decades since the APA thought that homosexuality was an illness or could be changed. While there is no conclusive evidence that homosexuality is purely genetic, the APA and other professional groups say that sexual orientation appears to be determined early in childhood and cannot be changed by therapy or other interventions.

> **TIP:** Many parents are racked with guilt when they find out their child is LGBTQ and are certain they must have done something wrong. This kind of thinking is unproductive. Focus your attention on accepting your child as he is, not on searching for a cause.

MYTH: Gays and lesbians are mentally ill.

FACT: In a 1957 landmark study, psychologist Dr. Evelyn Hooker proved that homosexual men and heterosexual men were not different from each other psychologically. Yet it wasn't until 1973 that the American Psychiatric Association removed homosexuality as a mental illness from the *Diagnostic and Statistical Manual*. In doing this, the APA made clear that homosexuals were as sound as heterosexuals. The following year, the American Psychological Association endorsed similar statements.

Since then, several studies have shown that gays and lesbians are just as mentally healthy as heterosexuals. The majority of the problems they develop, especially as teenagers, come from living in a hostile culture.

> **TIP:** If you are thinking of sending your child to a psychologist or minister to change his orientation, rethink this decision. Reparative therapy to change sexual orientation does not work and will only make him feel worse about himself and may cause depression, anxiety or self-detructive behavior. However, therapy may help your child communicate with you or resolve feelings of anger, confusion and sadness.

MYTH: Gays and lesbians try to convert or seduce others.

FACT: No one can convince or lure someone else into being gay or lesbian. Being gay or lesbian is not a choice nor is it catching. If your child is straight, he will not become gay or lesbian if he hangs out with a gay or lesbian friend or adult. There is no evidence that homosexuality is determined by association or any environmental factor.

> **TIP:** There are few positive role models for gay and lesbian teenagers. Encourage your child to seek out gay and lesbian adults, so they can fill that role. They can help your child feel less isolated and ashamed and give him someone to confide in. They can also be allies for you in reaching out to your child.

MYTHS ABOUT BISEXUALITY

People who are bisexual are attracted to both men and women. In a society that tends to put people in boxes as either gay or straight, someone who is bisexual can feel as if he has one foot in each but doesn't really fit into either.

MYTH: Bisexuals are really gay or lesbian.

FACT: They may or may not be. Some people who are gay or lesbian feel more comfortable saying they are bisexual initially, because they feel that will be more acceptable to others. Thus, they may come out as bisexual first and at a later date, say they are gay or lesbian. Conversely, many bisexuals first identify as gay or lesbian because our narrow gay/straight definitions leave little room for them to be who they really are. They later come out as bisexual when they find a label that is more authentic to them.

MYTH: Bisexuals are confused about their sexual identity.

FACT: Again, they may or may not be. Some teens have sex with boys and girls as a way of experimenting and testing until they find what feels right and natural for them. Others know they are truly attracted to both. Sometimes, we put the label "confused" on these adolescents because *we* are confused, more than because they might be.

MYTH: Bisexuals are sex-obsessed.

FACT: Because bisexuals are attracted to both men and women, people assume that they are having more sexual experiences and are more interested in sex than "normal" people. This is not necessarily true. Some have sexual experiences with men and women concurrently while others are with men or women at different times of their lives.

TIP: If your child appears to be bisexual, he may not know whether he's bi, gay or questioning his orientation. It's not helpful for you to demand, "Well, are you gay or not?" This simply pressures him unnecessarily, which will make him want to retreat to a place where no one is asking him for answers he may not yet have.

Try to let go of labels and just be there for him. He may want help, but not know how to ask for it. Use the skills we discussed in Chapter 1 to open up the channels of communication at home. But also have faith that he will work this out for himself because all children do.

MYTHS ABOUT QUESTIONING YOUTH

Teenagers who are questioning their sexual orientation are not sure whether they are LGBT or straight. Unable to seek support or advice from family or friends, they experience untold anguish trying to figure this out. Their questions and anxieties are endless. They're sure they are the only ones who feel so tormented and have no idea where to turn for information or for comfort.

Questioning teens aren't sure where they fit in. They cannot be pigeonholed into one of society's sexual orientation boxes and that makes them feel invisible.

Because they go unmentioned and forgotten, these teens often feel as if they don't exist. They are in limbo and alone. They tend to withdraw and silence their concerns because they feel that something must be wrong with them. Jason, the captain of the soccer team, has been wrestling with his sexual orientation. He became emotionally attached to Sam, his best friend who was gay. They had sex a few times but Jason felt something was not right. Originally, he thought he must be gay because he had had sex with a guy, but then he noticed how Sam watched the crowd: his eyes went guy, guy, guy. Jason's went girl, girl, girl. Did that mean he was straight? Was he naturally attracted to girls? But then how could he have had sex with Sam? Jason's head was swimming with questions.

Jason's parents probably don't know the turmoil he's going through. They see a child who is tense at home or who seems preoccupied. Walking the dog and watching television with his family are the last things on his mind.

Because teens who are questioning their orientation are virtually invisible, even myths about them go unmentioned, while almost everybody has heard a few myths about LGBT people. Here are a couple of myths that you should be aware of.

MYTH: Everyone knows what his or her orientation is. No one is really questioning it.

FACT: Questioning teens are a very real subgroup of teenagers. Because they are neither straight nor LGBT, they don't know where they fit in and society doesn't recognize them either. Yet because of their very precarious position, these teens are some of the most vulnerable and most in need of an understanding parent—not one who thinks they can fix their child.

MYTH: Questioning teens are really gay or lesbian.

FACT: They may or may not be. There are some who are honestly not sure. They may be bisexual and don't know what to make of it and are scared. They may be straight, but are experiencing a disconnect between their orientation and their behavior, like Mary, who adores her best friend Sally and only wants to be with her. She doesn't have sexual longings for her but thinks about her constantly. Mary now wonders whether that means she's really a lesbian.

Some questioning teens will turn out to be homosexual. They may know deep down on an unconscious level that they're LGBT but are so frightened that they refuse to accept what they know to be true. They just can't connect society's negative stereotypes of LGBT people with what they know about themselves. They are struggling to figure out who they are and where they fit in.

> **TIP:** Questioning youth desperately need their parents' attention. They are often silent and difficult to reach. But keep in mind: Every quiet child is not necessarily questioning his orientation. You know your child. If he has always been quiet, that may be his personality. But for youth who are normally talkative and outgoing, a "new" silence may cover up a secret, such as homosexuality. Questioning teens require special handling and will be discussed in full in Chapter 7.

SUGGESTIONS FOR PARENTS

Here are guidelines for creating a home that promotes each family member as a separate human being, who is loved and accepted for simply being himself.

Give your son a broad, positive view of masculinity

Today, our definition of masculinity is based on one-upmanship and rankings through sexual behavior and athletics. If you're good at both, then you're a real boy; the less interest you show in heterosexual sexual behavior and team athletics, the less of a man you are.

In *Cannibals and Christians*, Norman Mailer wrote: "Masculinity is not something given to you, or something you're born with, but something you gain and you gain by winning small battles with honor."

If that is your definition of masculinity, then perhaps you need to rethink it. Reflect on the men in your own life whom you have admired for reasons other than adherence to traditional male norms. Share those with your son and tell him why you admire them. Replace the antiquated notion of masculinity with one of honor and integrity: a good man does the right thing by other people.

To give your son a broader view of masculinity, begin with your own behavior. If you're a dad, you are his best role model. Let him see you cry when a relative dies or comfort your wife, daughter or son when they are troubled. Tell him about a male friend who did something caring or use examples from the newspaper or television to illustrate stereotypic male behavior as well as kindness in men. Fathers and mothers need to encourage and accept a wide range of behaviors from their son. Don't tell him, "Big boys don't cry" or "Keep a stiff upper lip." Let him show the same wide range of emotions that your daughter feels comfortable expressing.

Support your son in following his passion—whether it's drama, the arts or ice hockey—without a negative comment. Support these activities and let him know you accept him, whatever his interests. Tell him often, "I love you."

Teach your daughter a positive, healthy way of being a woman

In a world in which a young woman's currency is her appearance, sexual identity is a very valuable coin to spend. If you have the right sexual identity (straight) and you engage in the right sexual behaviors, you can think you are winning friends.

Help your daughter understand that her physical body is just one aspect of her whole self and that there are no wrong feelings (I'm attracted to girls) or wrong way to look (too heavy, too masculine). If you're a mother, counter the cultural messages by your own behavior: Don't obsess about your weight, diet constantly or count calories relentlessly. If you do, you're more likely to have a daughter who obsesses about food and her figure. If you're a dad, try telling her what a good job she did on her history paper or how well she played soccer, rather than complimenting her on her appearance— something you are trying to de-emphasize.

Encourage your daughter to develop her interests and talents in all different realms. Social activism (working in a soup kitchen, tutoring underprivileged kids, for example) will help broaden her worldview. She may become less preoccupied with trivial issues, like losing five pounds, when she meets, firsthand, people dealing with real survival issues.

Stop anti-LGBT rhetoric immediately

Not only can words hurt, but they create a closed atmosphere that conveys the message that you are only accepted and loved if you conform to certain rigid standards. One "liberal" parent confessed sheepishly that it took her a full year before she reacted to her sons telling each other, "Oh, you're so gay." A full year. The phrase was so ingrained in the culture that she didn't hear it and so didn't say a word.

When I was on the Governor's Commission in Massachusetts in the mid-1990s, young people overwhelmingly said that they were not so much bothered by the harassment as by the fact that the adults never did anything about it.

These issues arise every day—if you are sensitive to them. Here is a three-part process for handling anti-LGBT rhetoric in your home:

1. Note the behavior or comment and explain why it bothers you. You can say, "This kind of language really bothers me." Then explain why by saying either, "It's hurtful to people" or "It's based on the kind of thinking that puts other people down, which is something I never like to do."

2. Engage the other person in conversation about why he uses this language and why he thinks it's all right to do so. You can say, "I'm wondering if you've thought about the impact this kind of language has." Then let the other person talk.

   If a family member makes a comment, such as "I hate all queers," try to get more information behind the comment without being judgmental. You might ask, "What makes you say that?" Or "Why do you dislike gay people?" Once you hear him out, offer some facts. You might say that homosexuals have contributed much to society and name some prominent people who happen to be LGBT. If you have a personal relationship with someone who is a LGBT, you might talk about why this person has been important to you or why you admire her.

3. Draw the bottom line if the other person does not come around in your discussion. Say something similar to "This kind of talk is offensive to me and I don't want to hear it in the house again." If the other person realizes

she has been thoughtless and says, "You're right. I shouldn't talk like that," then you may not need to go to step three.

If you suspect that your child is LGBT, you have even more reason to stand up to offensive language. Don't worry that you'll embarrass him or even "out" him. My experience in talking with young people is that the one thing that hurts them the most is when biased comments go unchallenged. Most young people would rather feel embarrassed that you are standing up for them than feel that you don't care.

That doesn't mean you should take your stand no matter what. Do it in negotiation with your child, taking into account his wishes and the reality of the situation.

Keep in mind, too, that teens who are struggling with their orientation or are teased at school about being LGBT often "cover" by appearing macho and homophobic. They might be testing you to see where you stand on the issue.

If this discussion seems like a big leap for you, think about whether you allow teasing or cursing in your house. If you don't, then frame your stand on anti-LGBT talk within those values you hold dear. You don't allow offensive language in your home—period—and anti-LGBT language is offensive to you.

Be prepared that you may have to stand up again and again to anti-gay slurs and comments until the message gets across. It takes a long time to learn bigotry; it can take time to unlearn it. You may also have to confront relatives who grew up with or retain negative notions of homosexuality. Once you have decided on a zero-tolerance policy, it must apply to everyone in your home—whether your child has come out or not.

Walk the walk

If you want your home to be free of sexism and gender stereotypes, you need to practice what you preach. You can't control it when a grandmother tells your daughter that she's not "ladylike" when she does a headstand, but you can counter her comment by telling your daughter how well she's doing at gymnastics.

If you truly believe in gender equity, your actions will speak louder than your words. Try to get away from stereotypical male and female behavior so your children can see that men can be caring and sensitive and women can be tough and assertive. Being a positive role model can counteract some of the sexist and homophobic messages your children will encounter in school.

Of course, all of these changes take time and persistence. Many of them are far easier said than done. I am not saying that you should just "do it," but be intentional about the process of parenting, think through what kinds of messages you want to send your child and then act accordingly. It might mean you have to go out of your comfort zone and learn a new skill or behave in a new way, one that you were not prepared for by your parents or your upbringing. But parents do this all the time (how many of us are exactly like our parents?), and you will find your way.

Chapter Four

LGBTQ TEENS AND
THEIR FRIENDS

MY FRESHMAN YEAR of high school, Derek, a boy in my class, constantly made fun of me. He'd call me "faggot" and "gay lord" and point me out to the other kids. I was frightened of him. It didn't help that he was from a wealthy, prominent family and I was a child of a financially struggling single mom. He was also bigger than I was and the other kids were on his side; they always laughed when he taunted me. He was powerful and I was (I had started to see myself through his eyes) "a little fag." For all those reasons, I felt that I couldn't stand up for myself.

The fact that the harassment often happened with adults nearby who did nothing made me feel helpless, and disappointed. I expected adults, especially teachers, to stand up for me. But they never did.

One day when Derek had been making fun of me in English class, I decided I was going to beat him up after class. I sat in class, not listening to a word as the teacher droned. Meanwhile I was getting angrier and angrier. I guess I just snapped. I couldn't bear the teasing and humiliation any more and I didn't care what happened.

As we were leaving, I shoved Derek and knocked him down.

A bunch of desks fell over. I just stopped and looked at him, terrified by my actions, knowing he was going to beat me up. But he didn't. He just looked at me and left. No one had ever stood up to him before.

While on this one occasion I was able to stop the harassment, I endured it every day. Derek was the worst, but I lived in fear all day long. It began on the bus ride to school. I'd try to get the front seat, so I'd be as far as possible from the bullies in the back. I'd stare out of the window the whole time, pretending I was ignoring the kids' taunts. But they would still throw pencils and erasers at the back of my head. As soon as I got to school, I'd check in with my homeroom teacher and go to the library during homeroom so I didn't have to listen to the kids making fun of me.

I sat alone in the cafeteria for lunch.

I never told my mother what went on in school. I would never have involved her because I was humiliated. Telling my mom why I was being made fun of would have outed me to her and I was not about to do that. Also, I was a boy—boys were supposed to be able to take care of themselves and I couldn't. I didn't want to admit that either.

My mother was not the only one in the dark. You, too may be unaware of the constant and vicious teasing and torment experienced by teens who know they're LGBT, who are hiding their orientation or who are struggling with sexual identity issues.

While you may not be able to imagine this particular humiliation, you've had painful times in your childhood. We all have. Maybe you didn't have the right clothes, or you were overweight or you had a birthmark on your right arm. Every child has something she feels ashamed of at some point.

Take your most painful, humiliating moment in childhood and then multiply it a thousand times. Imagine it happening— not just one day—but every single day, in every class. That may very well be what your child is experiencing if she is LGBTQ.

This is a very serious matter. When students are abused or harassed, they have a tendency to minimize what's happening to them because they're embarrassed and ashamed. Sometimes they think it's their fault or they did something to "deserve" such treatment. Whatever your child is going through is probably much worse than what you're hearing—if you're hearing anything at all—because her own sense of shame and powerlessness often leads her to hide or minimize the extent of the abuse.

When your child is being targeted in any way—whether it is verbal, physical or sexual—you must get involved. You cannot excuse this behavior. You may think name-calling is not a big deal, but studies show that when verbal harassment goes unchallenged, it escalates to physical harassment. In almost every single case, when no one intervened, the bigotry increased and became a green light for further harassment.

Many parents think their child's school has no problems. That doesn't mean one doesn't exist or that one can't develop. In a focus group that GLSEN held in the summer of 2001 in Oak Park, Illinois, we found that parents were either ignorant about the amount of anti-LGBT bias in their schools or in near-total denial. They made statements, such as "gay students suffered 'teasing' but so do all kids" and that although anti-LGBT abuse was a national problem, it wasn't a "real problem" locally.

In this chapter, I'll give you a realistic look at what goes on among peers in classrooms, playing fields and locker rooms in the twenty-first century. I'll explore different kinds of bigotry, give you a better understanding of who the bigots and bullies are, and show you how to help your child handle harassment at school. I'll also give you specific suggestions for supporting your child when she comes home and tells you that she's been harassed, and offer ways to help fortify her to withstand the pressure of bigots.

HOW TEENS HIDE THEIR ORIENTATION

If you went into your child's school, you'd probably have a hard time figuring out who's LGBT, who's hiding and who's questioning her orientation. That's because these teens run the full gamut from students who are flunking out to those who are first in their class, from drug addicts to student council presidents.

But the vast majority have one thing in common: They are in pain.

They often don't show it. They may not give a sign of their distress to the outside world, but they are all going through internal chaos. One young man recalls his high school days, "When I would get teased about insignificant stuff, I would get upset. But when I started being teased about being 'so gay' you couldn't comprehend the degree of pain such teasing elicited."

The teasing was so mean, he says, that he hardened himself and let it ride over him—but not without it taking its toll: "I isolated myself from the situations where it was more prone to happen—places like team sports. These were really tough times internally." No one knew of his pain; he endured it alone.

Students choose different strategies to cope with their pain. These are all ways to avoid their true feelings or to compensate for being LGBTQ. Keep in mind that their behavior is not always conscious so they may not be aware of what they're doing. In the section that follows, I'll explain the ways youth who are LGBT or struggling with their sexuality—but are not out—hide their orientation. Each way is followed by a tip for handling what you see.

Heterosexual Activity

Many teens who are questioning or denying their orientation throw themselves into heterosexual activity, which may include promiscuity and pregnancy, as a way to divert their peers. They may also be trying to fool themselves or to prove to themselves that they couldn't possibly be LGBT. Look, they seem to be saying, I can't be LGBT. Look who I'm dating.

For some youth, simply dating the opposite sex is not "good enough." They engage in conspicuous and promiscuous heterosexual behavior, seeking to gain a "reputation" that will throw off their peers. Others are even more "out there" with their sexual escapades: they get pregnant or impregnate someone else.

According to the 1997 Massachusetts Youth Risk Behavior Survey, almost a quarter of gay, lesbian and bisexual students who have had intercourse have either been pregnant themselves or have gotten someone else pregnant. That's twice the percentage for sexually active straight students.* What better way to prove you're not LGBT than for a guy to be macho enough to impregnate someone or for a girl to be feminine enough to get pregnant?

TIP: Don't assume your daughter's straight because she always has a boyfriend or that your son is because he's a lady's man. Unfortunately, there is no guaranteed tip-off that things are not as they seem. That's what is so hard about this.

Focus on the behavior and probe why it's taking place rather than making assumptions.

If you're concerned about what seems like excessive sexual activity, discuss what is bothering you but don't focus on orientation. Follow these three steps:

1. Name or describe the behavior that concerns you without interpreting it
2. Ask what it means
3. See how she responds

If you try to explain the behavior, your child can focus on why your interpretation is wrong and avoid discussing her behavior.

For example, you could say to your daughter, "I noticed that you seem to have dated six different guys in the last two weeks.

continued on next page

---

* Lipkin, Arthur, p. 106.

That seems like an unusual number for such a short period of time." Then see where she takes it. If she says, "No, it's not," you could reply that you feel that it is and then list the reasons why someone may do that: "You know, in my experience, girls date a lot of guys for several reasons. They may have a desire to get to know many guys, they find different kinds of guys attractive, or they feel special when so many different guys are interested in them, or they want to show off the fact that they can attract so many different guys. I wonder if any or all of these are true for you." Let her take it from there. (Of course, if you have a son, you would change the genders in this dialogue.)

It may take several attempts for her to open up to you. Try again. Trust takes a while to build. If you do give up or get angry, that will confirm that you can't be trusted and that her initial assumption was right. Be patient and keep trying. If she shuts down, it's not a sign you did something wrong.

Overachievement

Financial writer Andrew Tobias coined the term "the best little boy in the world" in his book by the same name to characterize the lives of LGBTQ youth who are super-achievers. I'm a perfect example of that. I won awards, got elected to student leadership positions, and was the stereotypical "good kid." But all the while, I was still hurting inside, no matter how many APs I passed or how high I scored on my SATs.

Overachievers who are LGBT think like this: If I'm busy enough I don't have to deal with how I feel, and I can also try to win everyone's approval. Since I feel like I'm a bad person (because I'm LGBT), my achievements will make up for my being LGBT.

If I'm perfect, everybody will love me.

One young woman, who came out in college, recalls, "It's funny. I wasn't really interested in boys and I didn't have any interaction with them and I certainly didn't know why it was that I felt so different, but I was so busy in high school doing all this political activism stuff that I think that gave me an outlet for feeling different, because no one else was very politically active in high school. So everybody sort of looked at me funny for doing it."

A young man who came out to two teachers and a friend in high school remembers, "In high school I was very involved in student government, my classes and music. I also acted in theater productions. I remained in high esteem with my peers. I was known as extremely hardworking and fun—never seen at the wild parties or at those with the nerdy kids. I was very widely known."

Other youth compensate for being LGBT and for their low self esteem by being super-caregivers. They become the selfless friend who's always available, always ready to help, always willing to listen and commiserate.* By losing themselves in others' problems, they ignore their own needs and avoid their own feelings.

> **TIP:** You may take a lot of pride in your daughter's accomplishments. It may be tempting to let behavior that seems to meet or surpass the "norm" stay, but to do so may be to let a big problem fester.

Obsessive Behavior

Be on the lookout for obsessive behavior and for a child who seems exhausted and beleaguered. It's the relentlessness of the behavior that's a warning sign.

Such behavior is a way to cover pain and anxiety. If you can, separate your child from her achievements by asking yourself the following three questions:

---

* Lipkin, Arthur, p. 106

1. Does she seem happy?

2. Is she enjoying what she's doing?

3. Does she seem to be frantically trying to avoid something?

If you sense that she is avoiding, you could ask her, "What would happen if you couldn't do all these activities? How would you feel about yourself? What would you do with your time?" If you observe a sense of panic or a sense of loss when faced with this possibility, ask her what she thinks is prompting her feelings. You might say, "Sometimes people keep running or doing or bury themselves in school work or activities to avoid something. Is there anything that you might be running from?" See where she takes the discussion.

> **TIP:** Unfortunately, there is no way to know whether frantic, obsessive achieving behavior has a "sexual identity" component. You have to evaluate this behavior with everything else you know about your child and with everything else that is going on.

Distancing

When students use this technique, they attempt to get as far away as possible from anything that has to do with homosexuality. They avoid information about people who are LGBT, make homophobic comments and may even participate in harassment.* Psychologists call this reaction formation: warding off an unacceptable wish or impulse by adopting a trait that is diametrically opposed to it. Consider the guy who acts tough and gruff to cover his fears or the student who is frightened that he might be gay, and so becomes the loudest anti-LGBT bigot in the school.

* Lipkin, p. 106

Other students use diversionary tactics. Aaron, for example, diverts the conversation when asked about his relationships. He explains, "I sort of became a eunuch and I always avoided conversations where people started to talk about relationships. I'll help a friend with a relationship problem and then he'll go, 'Well, how about you?' Then, I'll go, 'Oh, did you see that article in *The New York Times?*' I'm pretty good at changing conversation if I don't want to talk about it. I learned that skill well—sort of avoiding those types of confrontations where I would have to talk about my relationships with anyone."

COMING OUT TO STRAIGHT FRIENDS

No doubt, your child has a lot of anxiety about coming out to her straight friends. You, too, may worry about how they'll react and whether they'll still like her and accept her. When straight teens befriend students who are LGBT, they themselves can become the target of bigotry. That may be another reason why your child is hesitant to

> **TIP:** An extreme reaction may be covering up some deeper feelings. Try to be sympathetic if your child uses distancing or diversionary tactics, and realize that more is going on than meets the eye. She's probably not ready to discuss what she's avoiding.
>
> I cannot give you a red flag to signal when your child is using these tactics. But you know when your child is trying to avoid you. Trust your intuition. You know your child.
>
> If you notice that your child is conspicuously uncomfortable with or troubled by something and you feel she might be amenable to discussion, point out the conspicuous behavior and ask why. For example, Aaron's father could have said, "I notice that whenever we discuss relationships, you bring up an article from *The New York Times*. I know you're an avid reader of the *Times*, but I wonder if anything else is going on for you?" See where he goes with it. If he says, "No. I just love quoting the *Times*," let it go. He's not ready to talk.

come out: her friends may be targeted for harassment, just for befriending her.

Matthew Schroeder, a twelve-year-old straight boy, is a case in point. In the spring of 2000, his parents filed a lawsuit in Toledo, Ohio claiming that the district did not protect their son from assaults and verbal abuse. The suit claims that two girls used sexual profanities and beat Matthew up on the school bus, damaging his kidney, because he was an outspoken supporter of LGBT rights and because his older brother is gay. The lawsuit is still pending.

There is an old saying that the gay movement began the day you came out of the closet and I think that's true for every LGBT teenager. What that means is that we each have to go through the process ourselves to understand it, and people tend to disbelieve the experiences of others until they experience the same thing.

They can hear stories of other teens and realize that coming out doesn't have to be a disaster, but many will remain convinced that they're going to lose all their friends until they personally come out, and don't. They are amazed that their friends stood by them, which they often do. That's because in many cases, by the time students come out, they've already gone through a number of stages, watching how their friends behave, and maneuvering themselves away from people who would not be accepting.

The reality is better than most teens expect it to be, but few believe that until they go through it themselves.

Jim's story will help you understand what your child may go through. In his last year of middle school, Jim passed a note during history class to one of his best (straight) friends telling him he was gay. After that, Jim told a few other people. At first he asked them not to say anything, because he didn't know how they'd react.

But then one of the guys whom he had asked not to tell spread the word that he was gay. Jim was shocked that people came up to him in the hall and asked him outright, "Are you gay?" At first Jim denied it, then he just brushed the question off with a "whatever" or "yeah." The following year, feeling more comfortable, he replied, "Yes, that's correct. I'm gay."

As far as Jim knew, all his friends were straight. "My friends obviously didn't care at all that I was gay. A lot of them were even to the point that they thought it was kind of cool or just fun or something to talk about. I didn't have any problems with my friends."

When he entered high school, students would pass him in the hall and point him out as "That's the freshman who's gay." Jim remembers how he felt. "I could tell just by the way people were acting towards me that it wasn't totally accepted," he says. "But this year I got to be friends with the 'popular people' and was more accepted. Now I don't think people care as much as they used to, because they've seen me act normal and I'm not like overly flaming—not that I think that's wrong. But they don't have a reason to be uncomfortable with me."

Jim was pleasantly surprised that his straight friends didn't drop him—as are most students. In my experience, though, girls tend to stand by their friends more often than boys do, which is why boys are more reluctant to come out in high school. Research has proven that boys are more homophobic than girls; the same holds true for men and women.

Parents can play an important role in helping their child come out to her friends. Although some may not see it as their place to do so, in fact, this could be one of the most wonderful supportive things you can do.

Here are four ways you can help prepare your child to come out to her straight friends:

1. Begin by reinforcing two important facts:
   • You can say, "Most of what I've read indicates that people judge you for more than just your sexual orienta-

tion. If people like you for so many other parts of who you are, it's doubtful that any one part of you is going to make them suddenly change their entire view of you."

- You can also add, "From everything I've been told, most gay teens do not lose their straight friends when they come out."

2. Although she probably won't be rejected, remind her that she doesn't have to stay in a situation that makes her miserable and that the situation she is in right now is not the only reality. You can say to your child, "You may have to change your course right now but that's okay. You'll probably have to change course many times over the span of your life, whether it's because of career shifts, death of loved ones or unexpected events in your life. The sooner you begin to understand how to deal with those changes and that they are not life ending, the better. I know it doesn't feel like it, but this is a great practice ground."

3. Remind your child what makes a true friend. You can say, "If your friends reject you because of your orientation, you have to wonder whether they were really your friends in the first place." And then go back to my last point and remind her again that if she loses these friends, she will find another group in which she feels comfortable.

4. Since many young people feel as if they will "never" make new friends, draw upon experiences your child has had, such as making new friends when she's moved, changed schools, or joined a new activity or sports team. This will help her see that she has done it before and she can do it again, if need be.

THE SCOURGE OF BIGOTRY

I know you're concerned about your child being in danger and you have every reason to be frightened about this. There is a real threat. But you don't want to become an alarmist. I am going to walk you through this minefield and fortify you with information, understanding and guidelines in three ways:

1. I'll give you the statistics so you understand the facts.

2. I'll put a personal face on the numbers.

3. I'll show you how to prepare your child to face her harassers at school and how to support her if she comes home and tells you she's been harassed at school.

Anti-LGBT bias takes many forms, from shunning to insults and name-calling to threats of violence to physical attacks. Whatever its form, it takes a tremendous toll psychologically, causing serious damage to young people's self-esteem. You may think that abuse only happens at other schools, that it could never happen in your school in "a good neighborhood." In fact, the tormenting that you'll read about crosses all racial, economic and cultural boundaries.

To make matters worse, many youth must cope with these affronts totally alone. While the parents of other minority youth, such as Blacks and Jews, have coped with racism or anti-Semitism themselves, LGBT youth are usually raised by straight parents, who have not experienced what their sons and daughters are going through.

As you read the section that follows, you will probably also wonder, where are the teachers and administrators? We will cover their position in detail in Chapter 9, but the fact is: the homophobia runs so deep that even the school staff may not get involved, or in their silence, condone the behavior.

For these reasons, I'm going to give you some graphic examples, so you know what it's like to be harassed on a daily basis or live with the fear of harassment.

While you're reading this, keep in mind that the best thing you can do to support your child is to continue working to create an open atmosphere at home. Keep the channels of communication open, so she feels free to share these frightening experiences with you and doesn't have to hide them in shame or suffer alone.

Just to give you an idea of how pervasive and constant anti-LGBT bias is, consider these statistics taken from GLSEN's 2001 National School Climate Survey that polled 904 LGBTQ youth from 48 states and the District of Columbia:

- 91 percent of youth reported that they frequently or often heard the expression "You're so gay."
- 85 percent heard homophobic remarks, such as "faggot," "dyke," or "queer."
- 42 percent reported experiences of physical harassment (being shoved, pushed, etc.).
- 21 percent reported being physically assaulted (being beaten, punched, kicked, etc.).

Sixty-eight percent of the students said they did not feel safe in their own schools because of their sexual orientation, and half felt unsafe because of their gender expression. In the following section, students reveal their experiences with different forms of anti-LGBT bigotry. Prepare yourself: These are not pleasant to read.

Shunning and Ostracism

It is not uncommon for other students to shun or ostracize LGBTQ young people. This is particularly true among girls (boys tend to be more physically aggressive). While they have no physical scars, the damage done is very real.

A high school student talks about her friend's experience of being at a party and accidentally revealing her sexual orientation to someone. "The next day the rest of school knew. Some of her friends ignored her; some people talked behind her back. Everywhere she went, she was treated differently by people although she was the same person."

Some LGBTQ students isolate themselves from their friends because they're afraid that someone will discover that they're LGBTQ or that they'll accidentally reveal something and become the target of abuse. One student said, "I was always an outcast at school. I ostracized myself from the rest of the world because I felt as if I could trust no one, not even my parents. The pressure of feeling so alone manifested in fits of manic depression, hysterical outbreaks, and eventually, suicidal tendencies."

Another student said, "I was depressed. Feeling alone and isolated from the rest of the world, I managed to fail three of my five majors that year."

Name-Calling

Verbal abuse is the most common form of harassment. Jared, who came out after transferring to a high school out of his district, recalls, "I was threatened just about every day—because I was a nerd. I wasn't out yet. People would threaten to beat me up all the time. It was just a very violent atmosphere there. You cannot be out and gay at that school. I really didn't have good days at all, because every day, I would be terrified of what would be around the corner—what bully would be there to call me names. A good day would be when nobody said something to me, which rarely happened. I would just get dirty looks. At least two or three times a day, someone would call me 'fag' or 'faggot.' "

The homophobia at Brigit's high school was more subtle but

just as pervasive. She was never called names herself but the name-calling surrounded her at school. It brought out all her insecurities. She recalls, "When I'm in an environment where people use the term 'gay' or 'faggot' as an insult, it really throws me off edge. Even though it's mostly boys using that against other boys, it makes me so nervous. It exacerbates my internalized homophobia and makes me uncomfortable."

Internalized homophobia affects many LGBT people in this way: They grow up in the same homophobic society as straight people. They take in all the negative messages about LGBT people that straight people do, but they also have a little voice in their head that constantly gives them negative messages about LGBT people—about themselves. So, they face external homophobia as well as internal homophobia.

In Brigit's situation, she was not just uncomfortable; she began to feel paranoid. "I was sure that when everyone saw me, they would think, 'Oh she's gay, I'm not going to talk to her.' It's kind of like the feeling that everyone is looking at you and disapproving of who you are and what you represent, and that people are going to judge you based on it. I don't know how much of it is rational and how much completely irrational, but it's a very real feeling that a lot of people experience. That can be really frightening, because it makes you think that your only options are either to go incognito and try to pass as straight or be like 'I'm gay, I'm gay, I'm gay,' which is especially difficult for someone like me who dates both men and women."

Threats of Violence

Students who are threatened with violence live on edge and in fear, because they never know when intimidation can turn to actual violence. Zoe Hart, a senior at Lincoln Sudbury, a school in an affluent suburb of Boston, testified at the Massachusetts Governor's Commission Hearings that "Last year at my high school, there was an incident which shocked everyone. Two female students were standing in the hall with their arms around each other. Students began to encircle them and yell profanities, until a group of thirty kids surrounded them." Living with the threat of violence can be frightening, unsettling and destabilizing. Even if the fears never become reality, students are highly aware of the threat, and often are completely debilitated and traumatized by it.

Like I did, they avoid certain activities and places where they think they'll be threatened. They stop talking in class, so they don't draw attention to themselves and engage in behaviors designed to hide their physical presence. They try to make themselves smaller and less visible, because they believe if they're seen, they'll get hurt. One common tactic is to let their hair hang in their face. Others include slumping in their seats, avoiding eye contact, and not talking in class.

Physical Assaults

Too often, though, threats *do* become reality. One in four LGBT high school students experiences physical assaults. There is no way they can feel safe in their school when they are the target of physical abuse. The following examples will give you a clue to what some students go through every day:

• A routine day for Andrew, fourteen, a small boy with straight hair and glasses, includes being body-slammed and shoved into chalkboards and dropped into trash cans head first by R., a bully who weighs more than 200 pounds. At a school dance, in the presence of chaperones and policemen, R. lifted Andrew above the crowd and ripped a pocket off his pants.*

• An eighteen-year-old gay student recalls, "I joined the drama club and the choir. I began the slow process of coming out

---

* *The New York Times Magazine*, August 22, 1999, p. 38

to my friends. This made things worse. I was spit upon, pushed, and ridiculed. One day I was sitting with some friends at lunch when, all of a sudden, a container filled with catsup came flying across the room and hit me."

• A gay male high school student speaks of the persecution he endured: "I just began hating myself more and more, as each year the hatred towards me grew and escalated from just simple name calling in elementary school to having persons in high school threaten to beat me up, being pushed and dragged around the ground, having hands slammed in lockers, and a number of other daily tortures."

WHO ARE THE BIGOTS AND THE BULLIES?

When I was growing up, my mother used to say, "Remember: When somebody points a finger at you, they have four fingers sticking back at them." I've always loved that because it reinforces what I want you to help your child understand: The bully has some kind of problem. He may be insecure, he may have fears that he's LGBT himself, or he may be trying to impress the "in" crowd.

This is the most important thing: Impress upon your child that it is the bully who has a problem—not her.

But bullies do not operate alone. They need an audience and they need acceptance for their behavior. They usually get both.

Psychologist Karen Franklin did an interesting study of anti-LGBT behavior among straight young adults. She found that ten percent reported physically assaulting or threatening people they believed were LGBT and almost 25 percent said they had called them names. More than half of the incidents occurred at school or in the workplace and while the perpetrators were part of a group. Among those who denied participating in any verbal or physical harassment, 23 percent had witnessed such incidents and presumably, did nothing.

This study fascinates me because we would like to portray hate crimes or sexual harassment as extreme, almost inexplicable behavior like lightning that strikes without warning or seeming cause. Or we delude ourselves into believing that such behavior is the work of one "bad apple." That is just not so. These are average kids. Research shows that severe harassment is at the end of a spectrum of behaviors, all of which were tolerated until they reach the extreme—rape or murder, as in the case of Matthew Shepard, the young gay man from Wyoming who was beaten to death.

People engage in testing behaviors as they move along a spectrum. Kids say, "That's so gay," or call someone a "faggot" or play "Smear the queer" in their gym class.* And no one intervenes or challenges them—until they cross a line and physically assault someone. (And sometimes, not even then.) Violence is the logical conclusion to a progression of behaviors that have been tolerated.

Part of how boys prove they are boys is by teasing girls and by picking on students who are LGBTQ. Often teens do this, because they are afraid of being labeled LGBT themselves or of becoming the victim if they don't engage in such behavior. These youth are learning to get away with bigotry. Whether it be toward LGBTQ people or women (or both), they are learning that it is acceptable behavior.

In a sense, we do youth a real disservice through hate crime laws or sexual harassment laws, because we allow them to engage in all the atrocious behavior until they hit a certain trip wire

---

* This is a football drill to teach students not to fumble the football. The "queer" is the one with the football. The goal is to hold onto the ball, no matter what. What better way to encourage boys to tackle someone hard than to tell them that he is queer?

and then we send them to jail. By the time they commit the rape, hate crime or sexual harassment, it is too late. They are just acting out behavior that has been tolerated for years, taking it to its logical extreme.

STOPPING THE CYCLE

You can help break this cycle. As we discussed earlier, if you hear anti-LGBT rhetoric of any kind and no matter how old the child, it is crucial that you make a strong statement, such as, "This kind of talk is offensive to me" or "I don't want to hear those words used in my house."

If you think your child is being bullied, ask her directly. Often children do not wish to tell their parents due to shame and embarrassment. Children also fear that the bullies will find out and retaliate if they tell, or that their parents will call the school and that will make things worse. The following four signs may mean your child is being bullied, but again they could also signify other things, so evaluate them in light of what else is going on with your child:

1. fear of going to school

2. lack of friends

3. missing belongings and torn clothing

4. increased fearfulness and anxiety

PREPARING YOUR CHILD TO HANDLE HARASSMENT AT SCHOOL

Many teens find ways to cope with harassment by trial and error. Jared trained himself to walk down the hall looking at the floor.

He says, "That's extremely hard for me to do because, I'm a very social person. I like to see who's here and say hi to this or that person. I like to look around and make eye contact with people but I couldn't."

He continues, "I totally ignored the bigots. That's why most of them stopped because I knew if I said something to them, it would egg them on. They would know that they got a reaction from me and so they could keep doing it. I wouldn't even turn around. I wouldn't even look at them. I would pretend that I hadn't heard anything. I didn't react at all outside, but inside of course I'm shaking, I'm nervous, my stomach is tensed up."

Todd chose another response method. When he was called names, he says, "I'd walk down the hall and someone would be like 'faggot' and I would look around and go, 'Yeah, Do you need something?' What are they going to do really?"

Todd and Jared seem strong and self-assured, or at least appear that way to their harassers. Do their parents know what goes on on a daily basis? They may not. If your son is already ashamed because people are telling him he's a little sissy, the last thing he wants to do is go home and say, "Hey, Mom, everybody is calling me sissy." He doesn't want you to point out to the school that everybody thinks he's a sissy because that will further shame him. So he may hide these experiences from you, as I did with my mother.

For this very reason, it's important that you teach your children how to protect themselves. If you have younger children, begin this process in grade school. If you're watching a television show and children are teasing each other or you overhear someone make fun of a friend at the mall, use that opportunity to bring up the subject. You can say something like, "I know kids can be mean to each other. They tease kids who are short or fat or different in any way. You may never experience this—and I hope you won't—but, just in case, I want you to know what to do. Let's talk for a few minutes about what to do if that ever happens to you." Then proceed to explain to her the three-step process for protecting herself:

1. Assess the safety factor. In some environments it is better to run than to fight. If you are in a hallway surrounded by the football team, that is not the time to fight back.
2. Estimate who is out there for you. Is there a sympathetic teacher, security guard or coach who can intervene on your behalf? If not, let it go.
3. Understand that this is not about you, that it's not your fault and that you have done nothing wrong. The other person—the bully—has the problem. Because there may not be sympathetic authorities or they may not be willing to intervene, it may not be safe for you to try to stand up for yourself. Remember that this is not about you. The bully is the one with the problem.

Use the following diagram to explain your points graphically:

	Unstructured Setting	Structured Setting
Supportive Authorities	Mixed Possibility for Success	High Possibility for Success
Unsupportive Authorities	Poorest Chance for Success	Mixed Possibility for Success

With your child, determine which quadrant realistically represents the situation at school. Keep in mind that she may be in different situations at different times, but this will give her guidelines for those variations. Then suggest that she follow the advice for that quadrant:

Top right: A structured setting, like a classroom, and the authority figures have shown themselves to be supportive: It is safe to talk back to your harasser.

Top left: An unstructured setting—a hallway, bus or bathroom— and the authorities have been responsive: Remove yourself from the threat immediately. Then approach the authorities and inform them of the threat and insist that something be done.

Bottom left: An unstructured site and the authorities of the school are not around or are not supportive: Remove yourself from the setting at once, report it to the school authorities or another organization, such as GLSEN, that can be an ally as you pressure the authorities.

Bottom right: A structured setting and the authorities have not shown themselves to be responsive: Approach the authorities and ask them to help.

If your child is in a safe place and there is a supportive authority figure around (upper right quadrant), what should she actually say to the bigot? Here are two rules of thumb to pass on to her:

1. If the harassment is directed towards you individually, respond directly to the harasser. If somebody says, "You faggot," you say, "I don't appreciate being called names like that."
2. If it's a kind of generic language not directed to you individually, focus on the language. If someone says, "Oh,

that's so gay," you can say, "Gosh, what's gay about that?" The purpose of this comment is to engage the harasser in a conversation, so you can help educate him.

Of course, it's ultimately the school's job to make sure young people get educated but in truth, the best person to educate the young is another young person. It's also a way to empower your child. So many LGBTQ youth feel that they have no power. Speaking up is a way to help your child regain control and lose the sense that she is a victim. If she does get some success from doing so, she can feel, "Wow, I can make a difference."

Remaining silent perpetuates a sense of powerlessness and helplessness that can be just as crippling as harassment: Helping your child learn she can stand up for herself (even if the behavior of others does not change, or at least not immediately) is invaluable in building her self-esteem.

But of course, under every circumstance and at all times, your child should assess her safety first. Then for direct harassment, respond directly to the harasser. For indirect harassment, question why that kind of language is being used.

WHEN YOUR HARASSED CHILD COMES HOME

No matter how much you want to and try to shield your child from harassment, there is always going to be some setting where you cannot protect her. Even if you have followed the guidelines in the last section to the letter, there may be a day when she will come home shaken and wounded from humiliation and alienation.

The following section will show you how to support her after she's been harassed while at the same time, give you ways to strengthen her psychologically, so she feels more powerful and can better withstand the taunts and torments of bullies in the future.

It will be hard for you to deal with harassment if you haven't already laid the groundwork for your child to be honest and open. If your child assumes you'll react badly, she's not going to share with you the real details of why she's getting harassed. She's going to try and hide them. Also if she doesn't feel very good about herself, she may feel that she deserves this, or it will bring further shame upon her if she tells you.

You're dealing with a double whammy. First of all, you may still be adjusting to the fact that your child is LGBTQ and now, you've just learned that she is getting hurt. Some parents in that situation will immediately—instead of blaming the school or her peers—blame the child and tell her that she needs to change how she behaves. They say things like, "If you'd just be a little more feminine, maybe they wouldn't single you out."

This is never a good idea. I know your intention is to protect your child but instead, it reinforces her sense of shame. You are echoing in her mind that she should feel this way, that maybe it's her fault. Parents react like this if they haven't worked through issue A (the fact your child is LGBTQ); then, they can't cope well with issue B, which is, how do I protect my child who's getting hurt?

As a parent, you absolutely must protect your child. LGBTQ youth need assurance that you're still their mom or dad and that if somebody tries to hurt them, you're still going to be there for them. We have found parents' involvement makes an enormous psychological impact with their children—even if it has little impact on the school. No matter what else fails, your child will know that at least you are fighting for her.

Here are practical suggestions for supporting a child who has been harassed. These are not necessarily in chronological order. Some steps will be done simultaneously. For example, while you are getting the facts you are also supporting her and empathizing with her

- Get the facts. Let her explain what happened to you. Just listen without interrupting. Use the listening skills we discussed in Chapter 1.

- Don't judge her or minimize what's happening. Never say, "Boys will be boys," or "Everyone gets teased sometimes," or "You have to learn how to handle these things." That will simply alienate her further, because you're denying her experience.

Keep in mind the old phrase, "Believe the impact." You may think she's overreacting, but you need to believe that whatever she's telling you is her reality. It may not make sense to you but if you doubt her, that's the surest way for her to think you don't "get" it. Telling her, "You shouldn't feel that way" is denying her reality and will only undermine your own credibility.

- Be honest with your child about the fact that you can't control what the school does, but tell her, "I'll be there for you and we're going to fight this together."

- Make sure the bottom line is clear. Say in one form or another, again and again, "Look I'm not going to stand for this. I'm not going to allow you to get hurt. I'm going to do everything in my power to stop it."

- Support her verbally by saying things like, "Yeah it sucks and it hurts," or "I'm sorry you're going through this."

- Review who her allies are. Ask her to name three people she trusts in the community or at school other than you who could help her. Give her the following suggestions:

> teacher
> guidance counselor
> coach
> clergy
> relative
> doctor
> youth group

- Focus on protecting her psychologically, by reinforcing her worth and by making sure she understands that the bully is the

one with the problem. She is not. Tell your child, "You don't deserve this. You did nothing to bring this on yourself. This is the
bully's problem."

• Talk about how you'll proceed. Make it clear that you're in
this together, but that your child will have a role in deciding what'
strategy you take. You can say to your child, "I'm willing to go to
school alone, I'm willing to go with you, or I'm willing to stand
outside the principal's door and you can go in alone. What do you
want to do?" Let her decide.

• Discuss practical strategies. For example, you can ask your
child, "Would it be easier if I picked you up from school rather
than have you ride the bus? Do you want to switch to another
homeroom? What would help you?"

• In Chapter 9, we'll discuss how to assess school policies, procedures and practices, and pursue legal protection, if
needed.

TO BE AUTHENTIC OR NOT

When your child sees bigotry around her at school every day or
has been harassed herself, she knows she has to make a decision
about whether to be authentic or whether to hide her orientation. A lot of teens are not successful in hiding their orientation,
because they're drawn to activities or behaviors that are gender
nonconforming, which automatically label them as LGBT. I
know these will probably sound like stereotypes to you, but
sometimes stereotypes are true to the reality.

If your daughter likes softball and chooses to be authentic, she 'may get called a lesbian, whether she is or not. If
she chooses to be inauthentic, she will miss out on doing the
things she likes. If your son is a naturally athletic boy and
chooses to go out for sports, he may feel he has to become a big
jock and engage in all the behaviors that are associated with
being a jock (excessive dating, bragging about his prowess, ridi-

culing people who are LGBT). Then no one will know he's LGBT.

I had that dilemma myself. I started getting picked on in the locker room when I was in junior high school. It was so bad that I had to quit playing sports. I made a choice to be inauthentic. I quit going. Today, I considered that decision one of the great tragedies of my growing up because I'd rather play sports than do just about anything. But at the time, I felt that I couldn't play, because I didn't want to be harassed anymore.

Teens come to a similar fork in the road: They either follow their authentic selves which can lead them to be harassed and ostracized, or they hide their orientation in hopes that they will not be persecuted or singled out. It's a tough choice: Are they authentic and do what they love, or do they give up their passions to avoid being harassed?

The results of an interesting retrospective study may help you guide your teen. Clinical and school psychologist Danny Carragher, in his doctoral dissertation for Hofstra University, found that closeted youth had lower self-esteem and engaged in more risky behavior than those who were out. Closeted youth had to monitor every detail of their behavior—how they walked, how they talked, how they dressed, whom they associated with—to make sure they weren't seen as LGBT. Constantly designing and redesigning their image and behavior requires enormous psychic energy. In addition, because they are not authentic, they cannot get support for who they really are.

In contrast, when LGBT youth are out, they are visible so others know who they are and can support them. They have the satisfaction of being true to themselves. Even if they are victimized, youth who are authentic feel better about themselves than those who are inauthentic.

Another factor at play here: Those teens who are authentic tend to have higher self-esteem and realize it's not they who have a problem; it's the bigot's problem. Teens who are inauthentic, on the other hand, tend to have lower self-esteem so they internalize the problem and blame themselves, thinking maybe they deserve to be picked on.

That doesn't mean, however, that every child should be authentic in every circumstance. Your child needs to determine what is right for her in any given situation. She probably has a better sense of her reality than you do since she's in the situation every day. Try not to deny what she knows is true, but do probe to see if her perception is based on fears or facts.

Here is a three-step process for handling situations like these:

1. Help your child understand the consequences of her actions. Probe a little bit with her and say, "Why do you think people are going to say you're a lesbian?" Or, "Gosh, what makes you say that?" Or, "Why do you think it's going to be so bad?" Your probing is to determine if there is truly a risk.

   Do try to help her separate fear from reality. But if, after that process, she's still convinced that the consequences she anticipates are real, you've got to acknowledge that and support her decision.

2. Help your child decide whether she wants to endure the consequences. Weigh the pros and cons. You can say to her. "If you do this, there will be this outcome. But if you don't do it, this may happen. Which of these would bother you more?"

   Then, go through the pros and cons with her, one by one. You might want to say to her at some point: "Throughout your whole life, you are going to face people who won't want you to do what you want to do, or be who you want to be. They will find various ways to try and dissuade you from that. If you let that run your life, you'll never do what you want to do or be who you want to be."

3. Support your child's decision. It may not be what you would have done or even what you want for her, but it's her choice. It's the decision she's comfortable with right now. Say to her in no uncertain terms, "Whatever you decide, I'm behind you 100 percent." Tell her that if she decides to play and the kids tease her, you're willing to go to school or do whatever she wants to stand up for her. If she prefers to handle the situation alone, respect her wishes. But do check in periodically to see how the strategy she has chosen is working, and if she wants to shift to a new one.

WHEN LGBTQ TEENS BAND TOGETHER

The link to other LGBTQ students and to LGBT culture is important in enhancing your child's self-esteem and identity. In her book, *Trauma and Recovery,* psychologist Judith Herman discusses the three steps in recovering from any trauma. Studies on trauma, from rape to child abuse, can give us clues to help young people traumatized by harassment. I have always believed that growing up LGBT in a homophobic society is a form of trauma, because the homophobia is continuous and you remain vulnerable for years.

The three steps are:

1. finding a safe space to talk about it

2. connecting with others who have experienced it

3. taking action to regain control

When your child connects with others who are LGBTQ, she will gain a sense of community and a feeling of belonging, which is important for any minority because they do not have the support of the larger community.

Do what you can to encourage her to meet other LGBT students, immerse herself in LGBT culture and join LGBT organizations. Here are some ways to offer concrete help:

- Offer to drive her to a meeting.
- Accompany her to a LGBT film festival if you feel ready.
- Mention web sites for LGBT youth.
- Point out the "gay and lesbian" or "gender studies" sections at the local bookstore.

When some students first come out, all they want to do is go to Gay Pride marches, read LGBT-themed books and see movies with LGBT stories. A lot of parents react with hostility to that and question their teens, asking them, "Before you liked all kinds of books and movies. Why now do you only like gay stuff?"

Many LGBT teens have had no exposure to LGBT culture prior to their coming out. They need to connect not only to other teens like themselves but to youth groups, political groups, cultural products like movies and books, and LGBT adults who can be role models. Your child may go through an "immersion" phase, because for so long she's had no access to LGBT culture and people. Now she may want nothing but access to those things, which is a natural reaction and a healthy part of her developing her own identity.

It makes a tremendous difference to teens who are striving to be authentic to receive the support of other students who are LGBT. Sometimes, just knowing that another LGBT student is around helps. Trish recalls her high school days and how having a role model helped crystalize her own thinking. "All my friends were pursuing relationships with men and everybody was talking about that and I never really wanted that. I couldn't figure out why I felt so differently than they did, but I knew that I was different," she remembers.

"It really didn't hit me until this woman who was a year ahead

of me came out in high school. I remember seeing her and thinking, that's what I want to be. I couldn't have told you why I identified with her. It was just I knew that what she had, I wanted. I
never talked to her or became friends with her, but I definitely
was in great admiration of her. She was my first role model, although she didn't know it."

For teens who are thinking about coming out or who have
just come out, actually getting to know another LGBT teen af-
firms their identity and lessens their isolation. Jared had seen
Julia around school and heard rumors that she had a girlfriend.
When his guidance counselor arranged for him to meet her, his
world opened up. "Even though I had met a couple of gay people
before her, I think the fact that she was someone in my everyday
life was a huge thing for me. If I wanted to see her, I just go to
school or call her, because she lives up the street. I didn't have to
go ten, fifteen, twenty minutes away to someone I never see. She
is the reason that I came out at school."

Seeing that Julia was comfortable in her identity made a difference for Jared. To him, everything was new and scary. "Being
gay wasn't a huge issue for her. It was just, this is what I am and
she talked about it very nonchalantly. Of course, for me at the
time this was a huge issue and I was terrified of being talked
about and even being seen with her because I knew what people
would think: If anyone's with Julia they must be gay. I remember
just feeling so alone before that and then after I met her, my
world changed."

Realizing what Julia did for him made him want to do the
same for other students. "You know what—kids need this," Jared
says. "I know there are other gay kids in this school who don't
know anyone and who don't know who to talk to. At least if they
have a visible sense that there is someone out there, they won't
feel so bad. I know that for a fact because Julia helped me. After
meeting her, I wanted to come out. Other students need to see
that they are not the only one."

Meeting LGBT students and adults and attending LGBT organizations or cultural events gives LGBTQ teens a sense of connection, which they have lacked for far too long and which is critical to their development of a positive identity. Because they don't have the support of the larger straight community, as straight teens do, the support and involvement in the LGBT community can give them a sense of belonging and normalize their experiences.

TAKING THE NEXT STEP

If you are aware that your child is being targeted for any reason, whether it is verbal, physical or sexual, you have an obligation to insist the school authorities—teachers, principal, superintendent—take action right away. Don't dismiss name calling or teasing. When verbal harassment goes unchallenged, bigotry increases and becomes a green light for further harassment. Chapter 9 will guide you, step by step, on how to become an advocate for your child. Involve her in this process because if you alone fight the battle for her, you reinforce the feeling she already has that she's a victim of abuse and has no power. You want to help her grow stronger so she can withstand assaults on her own.

Chapter Five

THE GAY, LESBIAN
AND BISEXUAL TEEN

IN MANY WAYS, I was the star of my family. I went to Harvard. I was a student council officer, a straight-A student and the debate team champion for my state.

But after I came out, everything changed.

A small event stands out in my memory as probably the most painful single incident I can remember. I came home from college sometime in the early eighties. I've always loved little kids, especially babies, and naturally gravitate towards playing with them at family gatherings. My brother had one daughter at the time who was about a year old. I was lying on the floor and she was sitting on my stomach and we were playing together. I had NPR on the radio and a story came on about AIDS.

There was kind of a pause in the conversation for just a second when the other people in the room, including my sister-in-law, realized what the story was about. I saw her look at me and her baby and, to her credit—I could see her physically restraining herself—she did not move. But I knew she wanted to snatch her child off my stomach. She was worried that I must have AIDS because I was gay, and somehow I was going to give it to her child.

I don't know if anyone else was even aware of what happened. I doubt my sister-in-law would remember the incident today, but it was significant to me, because I went from playing the role I usually play in the family—the fun uncle—to being a social outcast, a danger to the children in the family—even momentarily.

This is the very reason many LGBTQ youth are afraid to come out: They fear that their role in the family is going to be completely compromised and ruined. They fear they'll go from being loved or favored to no longer being accepted and adored.

And it's not an unrealistic fear.

In this chapter, we'll look at your child's coming-out process as well as your own. I'll show you how to cope if you and your child are at very different places or if you and your spouse seem at odds. I'll give you advice for making your child's process smoother and for supporting her throughout. I'll also discuss how to break the news to family members and how to find support for yourself. When you finish reading this chapter, you should have a blueprint for helping your LGBT child come out.

A WARNING ABOUT THESE MODELS

In the sections that follow, I'm going to present a parent and child's model for coming out. Both of these are based on developmental models that chart the stages that a child and parent typically go through as they progress in awareness and understanding. While helpful in giving us a framework, both these models have serious flaws. One size does not fit all. There are too many variables in real life. Such factors as race, religion, ethnicity, age of parents, age of child, and birth order of child (parents of a first-born typically have a harder time than those coping with a second or third child) all play a part.

Keep in mind, too, that these stages are not linear. People do not progress logically step by step, from one stage to the next.

You may move back and forth between stages, stay in two stages at once, or begin your process at stage three. Feelings are not locked into stages either. Many emotions occur simultaneously, or they may shift within a single day or even within the hour.

Your process and your child's may bear little resemblance to the ones offered here, but these models do give us a basis for comparison. It helps us understand that there is a process at work, and we're not alone in experiencing it.

A MODEL FOR COMING OUT

Everyone—whether they are LGBTQ or straight—goes through a process of developing a sexual identity. Heterosexuals don't recognize themselves as having a heterosexual identity because that's what's expected of them. Just as very few White people think of themselves as White, by comparison, most Black people are highly aware that they are Black, as a result of the covert and overt hurdles they face daily because of their race. So it is with people who are LGBT.

Clinical and developmental psychologists first proposed coming-out models over two decades ago. These describe the steps that individuals take from first awareness of same sex attraction to accepting and integrating a new identity into their personality and their life. I follow what is called a Mega-Model, which merges the models of three scholars of lesbian/gay identity development. The best way for me to describe the five stages is to illustrate each with an anecdote from my own life. The stages are:

1. Pre-Sexuality
   Many LGBT youth talk about how they felt different from their peers from a young age. Although this sounds simplistic, it is a factor: Girls often have an interest in sports when all their friends are playing with dolls, and

boys prefer to cook with their mothers or play with the girls, rather than hit a baseball. I remember in third grade we were asked to bring in carpet remnants to nap on. My best friend was a girl so I put my rug next to hers. This created such a ruckus with the boys that the next day, wanting to be accepted, I moved to their side. They teased me relentlessly. I had crossed the boundary—I had sat on the girl's side. I was no longer one of the boys and wasn't allowed to sit with them.

2. Identity Questioning

Youth begin to question whether they could be LGBT and whether stereotypes about LGBT people fit them. They often distance themselves from their family and straight friends in the process. They avoid typical LGBT behaviors or will obsessively date the opposite sex—to prove they're straight. In junior high, I developed a grid in which I graded the body parts of the cutest guys in my class, ranking them from one to ten on arms, chest, thighs, etc. I told myself I did this so I knew what a perfect body would look like. In truth, I was attracted to them but I denied the sexual component and blocked out any information that would indicate I was gay.

3. Coming Out

Teens move from tolerating to accepting their identity and come out to immediate family and close friends. Once I had come out, I wanted to talk about it all the time. My sophomore year of college, I'd meet someone and say, "Hi, I'm Kevin Jennings. I'm gay." I worked this information into every conversation. I was obsessed with talking about being gay because for so long, I couldn't say a word. I also immersed myself in LGBT culture and only listened to music by LGBT groups.

4. Pride

Teens move beyond acceptance when they feel good about this part of themselves and take pride in their

identity. I used to be a totally preppy kid who had tons of
Izod shirts. When I came out in college, I immediately
switched to a kind of new wave punk appearance. I wore
a thin little tie and a black blazer I had bought at a rum-
mage sale, and had about a half a pound of gel in my
hair. My new appearance was very much associated with
my new pride in being gay. To me, being gay meant that
you were avant-garde and funky, so I dressed the part.

5. Post-Sexuality

At this point teens have integrated their homosexuality
as one part of their identity. They move beyond thinking
of themselves as an LGBT person to a person who is
LGBT as well as funny, smart, talented, etc. There is no
longer a need to dress or act a certain way. I am a natural
athlete, yet once I came out, I avoided athletics because
I thought it wasn't "gay." Now that I have integrated my
identity, however, I feel comfortable saying, "I play ice
hockey and I'm also gay." I don't need to fit stereotypes. I
can just be me.

As a parent you may not be aware that your child is even on
such a path. Most young people don't come out until they reach
stage 3 or 4, but it's important for you to be aware of the process
so that you understand where your child has come from by the
time you receive the news.

A PARENT'S PROCESS

When Terri's son, Michael, put his hands on her shoulders,
looked her in the eyes and said, "Mom, I'm gay," Terri thought
her whole world had collapsed. She had thought he was coming
over to tell her he was getting engaged to his girlfriend of four
years. Terri was inconsolable for weeks.

Anne, on the other hand, had suspicions that her daughter Jane might be a lesbian. She never dated, didn't seem interested in boys and was very involved in feminist politics. When Jane said, "Mom, I have something to tell you. I'm tired of lying to you. I'm a lesbian," Anne was relieved to learn why Jane had become so distant but she was upset, too. She cried every day as she drove to work. Then she'd sit in the parking lot, dry her eyes, freshen her makeup, and steel herself to go in, putting up a facade that everything was fine.

Like these two mothers (they are usually told before fathers), you will have your own feelings and your own process of coming to terms with the fact that your child is LGBT. You might be devastated, as Terri was. Or you might feel relieved to have your suspicions confirmed, like Anne, and not have to tap dance around the issue anymore, but also feel disappointed that any hope for heterosexuality is gone. It is a rare parent who can immediately and wholeheartedly embrace her child when she comes out.

More typically, parents go through a series of steps to come to terms with the fact that they have an LGBT child. Traditionally, we have understood this through the lens of a process based on the work of psychiatrist Elisabeth Kübler-Ross's stages of coming to terms with a death, which she explored in her landmark book, *On Death and Dying*. This model has been applied in recent years to people facing illness and painful events.

There are obvious shortcomings with applying a model about something as shocking and tragic as death to how parents react to the news that their child is LGBT. It assumes, for instance, that the news comes as a surprise to the parent (it often isn't a surprise at all) or that the parent always views being LBGT as tragic (many parents do not).

But many parents *do* experience a kind of grieving for the "loss" of their heterosexual child as well as their own loss—of the hopes and dreams they had for a traditional life for their child—

after learning their child is LGBT. They may also mourn their lack of grandchildren and their perceived inability to be a grandparent. Parents who blame themselves for producing an LGBT child, who had previously thought they were doing a good job, grieve for their lack of success as a parent.

It may take months or even years to work through all these complicated feelings and stages. It took Terri four years to get to the point of not caring what other people would think. Anne, who has known for thirteen years now, feels totally accepting of her daughter and her partner, although she is still bothered that she might not have grandchildren. (And in turn, her daughter may feel guilty for disappointing her mother by not giving her the grandchildren she wants.)

There is no right or wrong way to progress. Everyone has her own process. Use these stages as a guide; they are not an absolute. You might skip a stage, reverse the order or never enter one at all. Whatever you're feeling, rest assured that you cannot deny, avoid or repress your emotions—you're going to have to deal with them, and that is a complicated process.

But keep this thought in mind: Many other parents have gone through the same process and have come out with stronger relationships with their children because their child came out. You can, too.

Here is a capsule definition of the stages:

Denial is a typical response when parents first learn that their child is LGBT. Some of their comments include:

"It's just a phase. You don't know what you want."

"Are you sure?"

"You're just experimenting. That's all."

According to a national survey, most LGBT people wait an average of four and a half years after knowing their orientation before they tell others; so by the time they come out, they are sure and they do know.

Anger, often masked as fear, hurt and disappointment, surfaces in many ways. Parents are furious that their calm, "normal" life has been shattered with the news and many make hurtful comments to their child, or blame an LGBT friend or partner for seducing their child.

Bargaining takes many forms. Some parents make pacts with God or the spirits or promise to reform their life. Some urge their child not to tell anyone or bring it up again, hoping it will go away in the meantime.

Depression often follows when parents learn their child is LGBT. Although many LGBT people end up having children, some parents immediately focus on the "fact" that they are not going to have grandchildren as a major disappointment. Parents also worry that life will be hard for their child and that she will have to endure discrimination. And some parents turn on themselves, feeling that they must have done something wrong to cause this.

Acceptance results when parents realize their child is happier now that she's out; the child has a new place in the family, which now has more honesty and more open lines of communication.

Elisabeth Kübler-Ross's stages end here, which I consider a flaw when her model is applied to coming to terms with an LGBT child. I believe parents move beyond acceptance (to borrow a page from their child's stages) to two more stages:

Pride

These are often the PFLAG moms who are fired up for their children and really "out there." Their children are sometimes at the level of synthesis and are kind of embarrassed by their parents and wish they'd tone down. Think of Michael's mom in the Showtime series *Queer as Folk,* who is much more of an activist than her son.

Synthesis

The final stage occurs for parents when their child becomes more than just their LGBT child. The only time I saw Matthew

Shepard's father, Dennis, get angry was at a meeting was when someone referred to Matthew as his gay son. Dennis Shepard was furious and said, "He was not my gay son. He was my son who was gay and who was smart and who was talented and who was kind." Dennis Shepard was at the end of the developmental spectrum.

In fact, by the time Matthew came out to his parents, they were way beyond denial. They had known for years that they had a gay son. This family illustrates the shortcomings of the Kübler-Ross model, which assumes every parent is clueless, has no self-awareness and the minute she finds out she is shocked and horrified. That is just not true for a lot of parents.

BLENDING YOUR PROCESSES

You have your own process and move at your own speed and at your own pace, as does your child. In most cases, you and your child will not be at the same point at the same time.

It is not necessary, or a good idea, for you to share all your ups and downs or all your mood fluctuations with your child. Your moods will influence her. She has enough to cope with with her own process and with interactions and anti-LGBT bias at school. Here are four steps I recommend you follow if you and your child are at different points:

1. Acknowledge that you are behind your child in her process. If your child wants you to march in the Gay Pride parade, you can say to her, "I just can't march yet. Let me tell you why: it doesn't mean that I don't love you but I'm going through a process too and I'm hoping someday I'll be able to go to the pride march with you. But right now, I'm just uncomfortable." This statement lets your child know that this is your issue and you know it's your issue. It helps the young person understand that

it's not about her. Talking about it will keep the relationship intact and honors both of your processes.

2. Pledge to work on it. Tell your child what you feel you
need to do to enable you to move ahead. For example,
you might say, "I feel as though I need to read a couple
more books by parents of gay children" or "I want to go to
PFLAG meetings for a few months, then I think I'll be
ready to join you" or "I need to do some more soul
searching. There are a couple of things I need to work
out before I feel ready to accompany you." If your child
continues to press you, you can say, "I'm doing the best I
can right now. Please be patient with me."

3. Give yourself the space and time to do the necessary
work. Make this a priority in your schedule. Write it into
your daily calendar if you need to. Then, proceed to do
whatever you have pledged to do, whether it's reading,
talking with other parents, or spending time alone reflecting.

4. Give your child updates so she can tell that you're ac-
tively working to remedy the situation. Mention a point
you read in a book or tell her something you learned
from another parent, so she sees that you're serious
about closing the gap between you.

Occasionally, parents are actually ahead of their children.
These parents are the ones who want to go to the gay pride parade
and the child is embarrassed by the sometimes-outrageous nature of the parade and doesn't want her parents to see it. If you're
such a parent, I would say to you, "Don't push it. Please back off."

WHAT REALLY MATTERS

While an awareness of these stages can be comforting to parents, they only tell part of the whole story. The Kübler-Ross

model assumes that every single parent shares the same attitude, the same degree of self-awareness and the same kind of relationship with her child. I have found that two factors are most important in determining your reaction to your child's coming-out:

1. the quality of your relationship with your child

2. your self-awareness, attitudes and openness toward LGBTQ people.

If you have a comfortable, relaxed relationship with your child and have done the self-reflection exercises, you will handle this situation well. The following diagram will help you determine where you are in relation to these two areas and how this process will unfold for you.

	Relationship with Your Child	
	Worse	Better
Self-Aware	Some Difficulty with Adjusting	Greatest Possibility for a Smooth Adjustment
Not Self-Aware	Greatest Difficulty with a Smooth Adjustment	Some Difficulty with Adjusting

Degree of Self-Awareness (label at left, between Self-Aware and Not Self-Aware rows)

BREAKING THE ICE

You may wish this whole "gay thing," as one parent put it, would go away. That's not uncommon among parents of LGBT youth.

But not talking about your child's orientation will only change how your child feels about it and expresses it. It won't change her orientation. Denying the subject will only make it harder for her to come out and create more distance in your relationship.

Even if you don't feel like it, you must break the ice.

Before teens come out, they often test their parents to see where they stand. One child may start watching *Will and Grace* to see if you comment, or may ask what you think of Will or Jack. Another may join a gay-straight alliance at school and start talking about the meetings at home.

If your child asks you what you would do if your new neighbors were two gay men, for example, the following responses send a red light and tell her that you're not interested in talking:

- Ignore the question and continue with what you're doing or walk out of the room.
- Dismiss the question with a comment like, "That would never happen in a neighborhood like this."
- Make a direct negative comment, such as "I would not want gays living that close to me."
- Make more subtle comments, such as "I guess it'd be OK," or "That's their business," or "That's more information than I need to know."

In contrast, the following responses send a green light:

- Put down whatever you are doing, look at her and respond by saying something like, "I'd have no problem with gay neighbors. How would you feel?"
- Say "I'd judge them like anyone else who moved in, basically on how good a neighbor they are. That's more important to me than if they are gay or straight."
- Make a more positive comment such as, "I'd

> treat them like I do all our new neighbors. I'd go
> over and welcome them and bring them a cake or
> a plant, or invite them to dinner."

If none of these comments matches how you truly feel, you might say, "Wow, I don't know how I'd feel. I'll have to think about that." It's important to say things that are true to you. Young people can tell when their parents are being insincere.

If your child gets a green light, she will continue opening the door a little bit more. Until she is ready for an open dialogue, try to reinforce every sign that she gives in a positive way. It lets her know it's okay to continue and that the light is still green.

Brigit remembers how important her mother's little hint was to her, because they had not talked openly about her being a lesbian. "At the beginning of the year my mom asked me how things were going at school and I was like, 'Well, there is this girl named Pam that I've been hanging out with almost all the time.' And she sort of smiled. My ex-girlfriend was also named Pam, and my mom started smiling and said, 'You really like girls named Pam, don't you?' That was a little moment. It's really silly but it's acknowledging it even if you're not openly talking about it." Her mother's smile, a non-verbal confirmation, was particularly encouraging.

To make it even easier for your child to open up and come out, give her hints that you know or suspect in a non-direct way. One girl said, "A lot of times kids are waiting for their parents to bring it up or for signals from their parents that they know something. If the parents are not giving those signs, usually kids assume that it's not okay to talk."

In addition to my suggestions in Chapter 1 for creating an open atmosphere, here are four other ways you can create a climate of affirmation and acceptance in which your child will want to come out:

1. Apologize for past insensitivities, such as homophobic jokes or language. If you realize that you've made an offensive comment, you can say, "You know, I was thinking about something I said the other day and I'm bothered about it. I didn't mean . . . when I said . . ."

2. If you've had a positive personal experience with someone who's LGBT, relate that in a natural way. If a colleague at work is LGBT, try to bring that fact into the conversation so your child knows that you're open to all kinds of people. You might say, "At lunch today we were discussing annoying habits of our partners and after I said . . . about Dad, Jim, who's gay, talked about issues with his partner."

3. Initiate conversations about sexuality that show your openness to people who are LGBT. Try to do this naturally when you discuss the facts of life. Make sure to include from time to time the phrase, "whether you're gay or straight," in your discussions. For example, when discussing STDs, you might say, "Whether you're gay or straight, you need to protect yourself."

4. Bring a dialogue about LGBT issues into your home. When you are discussing political issues or current events at the dinner table, make a point to bring up LGBT-related issues, such as the Boy Scouts' anti-gay policy, gays in the military or same-sex marriage. You can begin by saying, "I was outraged when I read in the paper this morning that . . ." or "I've been reading about these gay-straight alliances in high schools: Do they have one at your school? Is it needed? Do you think it would be a good thing?"

These conversations are important, whether or not your child responds the way you want her to. They show that you're making the effort and that you care. One day she'll be thankful for that.

COMING OUT AS GAY OR LESBIAN

You may have suspected for a long time that something was bothering your child or that she was distancing herself from the family and couldn't figure out what was going on. Even though same-sex attractions may be foreign to you or make you uncomfortable, value the disclosure: It gives you an explanation for your child's behavior and can put other fears to rest.

You will set an inviting stage for your child to come out if you continue to keep the green light on by sending hints yourself or by responding in a positive way to each of your child's clues or tests. Ideally, she will initiate a direct conversation in person, but some teens do come out over the phone or by letter, or sometimes school officials, friends or unexpected circumstances may "out" a child.

Of course, too much positive feedback can be intrusive and off-putting. David, Todd's father, overheard a telephone conversation late one night in the summer before ninth grade. Todd had a crush on a guy and told a friend, "Gosh, I really hope that he's gay." His father picked up the phone, heard enough, and told him to get off the phone. Todd recalls, "I was freaking out the whole next day. Then my dad said he needed my help to move something at his office."

David took Todd to his office, sat him down and said, "I heard part of your phone call last night." Immediately Todd said, "It's just a phase."

David said, "Well, just a minute. I just want you to know that whatever you decide I'm going to be behind you 100 percent."

Todd was shocked. "I did not expect that," he recalls. "I still didn't know how to take that and I really didn't want to talk to my dad about stuff like that. I told him I'd rather not talk about it. He was like, 'Okay, but when you feel like talking about it, just let me know. Whatever you choose I'll stand behind you as long as you know that's what you want.' I was like, 'I don't really know, so let's not talk about it.'"

A couple of weeks later, Todd told his dad he decided that he was going to be celibate and not date guys or girls. Todd recalls, "We were standing outside the car about to get in and he pounded his hand on top of the car and said, " 'That's just stupid. That is the dumbest thing I've ever heard. I'd rather you be gay than celibate. That doesn't make any sense.' After that I was like, 'Let's not talk about it again.' "

Todd wanted to be private yet at the same time, he was still talking to his dad about his sexuality. David went overboard in his reaction—he was way ahead of Todd in the process. Not only did he completely accept his son's homosexuality from the very beginning but he was almost insistent—banging his hand on the top of the car—that Todd accept it too. This aggressive approach would not work for everyone. Another child may have been intimidated by such antics and stop talking to his dad altogether.

Todd's situation illustrates how you need to proceed with caution, be sensitive to your child's personality and tune in to her feelings at every step of the way. By the time your child is fourteen or fifteen years old, you have a pretty good sense of her basic personality, and through trial and error, have figured out how to communicate with her. Chances are, she is going to handle this problem just as she's handled every other problem in her life. The following three suggestions may help you as well:

1. Reflect on how you've handled difficult situations in the past: What have you done that has worked with your child? How did you break the news about a divorce or a death in the family? Do it now.
2. If you don't know or haven't found anything that has worked in the past, ask other parents whose child has a personality similar to yours for advice. You can say, "I'm having a hard time getting Susan to talk to me. You and Jane seem close. What have you done to get Jane to talk to you?"
3. Notice if there are other adults—teachers, grandpar-

ents, older siblings—whom she seems to communicate well with. Then ask them by saying something like: "I noticed that you and Susan have a great relationship and Susan and I don't. I'm wondering if there is anything that you could tell me, based on your experience, that could help me learn how to talk better to Susan."

When your child comes out to you, there are several important things you need to do. As with all serious conversations, you'll begin by putting down whatever you're doing and give her your undivided attention. Then:

• Let her do the majority of the talking. Just listen. There's an old rule of thumb in job interviews that you should let the candidate do 70 percent of the talking. Your child deserves at least as much air time.

• Encourage her to keep talking by saying, "Tell me more," "How do you feel about that?" or "I see."

• If you're having a hard time with the news, be upfront and say, "This is difficult for me. I need time, but I know this is not going to make a difference in our relationship in the long run. You'll always be my child and I'll always love you."

• If you can, tell your child, "I love you," and "I'm proud of who you are." She may fear that you don't love her in the same way since she's come out. Your comments will reassure her.

COMING OUT AS A BISEXUAL

As discussed in Chapter 2, there are people along the sexuality continuum who are at varying degrees of bisexuality:

• those who are primarily homosexual who have some opposite-sex attractions

- those who are basically heterosexual with some same-sex attractions
- those who float along the middle range.

Some teens who say they are bisexual in high school will remain bisexual. Some will join the heterosexual camp later and some will eventually come out as gay or lesbian. The reverse is also true, in that some teens who say they're straight will later identify as gay or lesbian, and some who say they're gay or lesbian will later come out as bisexual.

These are some of the issues that teens who are bisexual face:

- They feel as though they don't fit in either the lesbian/gay or straight communities yet feel constant pressure to join one camp or the other, depending on the gender of their current partner.

There was a young bi woman on our staff who always felt a part of the office's LGBT community. Yet when she decided to marry her male partner, the office felt angry and betrayed. They felt as though she were no longer one of them. In some ways she wasn't, as her relationship was now recognized in law in a way that her LGBT colleagues' relationships were not. But her feeling of exclusion and loss was hardly mitigated by that cold legal fact.

- People who are bisexual must also contend with enormous bias against them for supposedly being promiscuous. The bisexual community has even poked fun at this stereotype by launching a magazine called *Anything that Moves* that parodies some people's beliefs about bisexuals' willingness to engage in indiscriminate sexual behavior. Teenage girls, in particular, come under tremendous pressure from boys because there is a perception that bi girls are hyper-sexual and thus sexually available all the time. Of course, this is not true, but that's the image because they are attracted to boys and girls.

Bethea identified herself as bisexual all through high school. She explains how that came about. "I joined the gay-straight alliance when I was in eighth grade. I knew I was straight, but I had decided that gay rights was going to be my own little movement or whatever. I think unconsciously it was because I was queer, but I didn't know it yet.

"I had a huge crush on this older girl at the school. I really didn't identify it as a crush at first. It was more that I wanted to be like her because she was politically active and cool. I was like, wow, I want to be just like her. A friend of mine pointed out, 'That's not what you want: you want to be *with* her.' I sort of became aware that maybe she was right. Then I met a student who identified herself as bisexual. Meeting her was validating just because I thought, 'Hey, I could like maybe use that word to describe myself.'"

Bethea had a girlfriend in tenth and eleventh grade. During her senior year of high school she dated men and women, and continued to think of herself as bisexual. Today at twenty-two, Bethea has dropped the bisexual label and identifies herself as a lesbian. Looking back, she says, "I think the label was valid in high school and I don't think I was kidding myself or anything. It's a tricky subject because now I don't think I'd ever date men but I would have sexual relationships with them. It's a very different thing when I'm with a man and with a woman."

Some people, like Bethea, just don't fit neatly into a gay/straight pigeonhole.

It's a natural human desire to put others—and ourselves—in boxes so that we can understand them. People want to put themselves in a category that makes sense, particularly when the categories are as clearly defined as they are today. The biggest casualty of this are the bisexual teens.

If your child has come out to you as a bisexual, all the parenting guidelines in this chapter apply to your situation as well. Here are two additional pointers:

1. **Don't jump to conclusions.** These are the words your child is using to identify herself. It's the language she's comfortable with right now. She's not "really gay": she's whatever she is saying she is.

2. **Accept the label she is using and don't question her about it.** Nonetheless, understand that some people do move along the continuum as they develop a greater understanding of themselves.

WHEN PARENTS ARE AT ODDS

You and your spouse are totally different people. You each have your own personality, background, and biases and prejudices. You each have a different relationship with your child. It is unusual for a child to have an equally strong relationship with both parents; most children feel closer to one parent. It is also more common for husbands and wives to respond to their child's disclosure differently and to accept it at different rates.

A year and a half after David's outburst, Todd began, little by little, talking to his dad. When he had his first boyfriend his senior year in high school, he told him about it. He didn't come out to his mother Mary until his junior year of college. His father told him she couldn't handle it. She would drop threatening hints, like "If I ever found out you were gay, I don't know what I'd do." Her comments sent Todd a red light for a long time.

When it became obvious that Todd had a serious boyfriend in college, Mary asked him if they were dating. Todd recalls her reaction: "She was really upset about it. She threw a fit. She didn't know how to handle it. She's like, 'Well, I always wanted you to have your own family.' I was like, 'Well, I will have *that* but I'll just be with a guy.' She didn't like that. She didn't know how she would ever talk to her friends about it."

In Todd's family, his dad continued to express total support. Todd says he and his dad are best friends today and they can discuss anything. It took his mother much longer to accept the situation. She didn't tell her friends for several years. She was too ashamed, and she kept hoping that he would change and all the turmoil would go away.

Today, five years later, Mary says, "I've accepted it. It's the best it can be. But I wish he weren't gay because it's a harder life and I'll wish that till the day I die."

In another family, both parents learned that their daughter was a lesbian at the same time, yet they had totally different reactions as well. Elise remembers, "Jim and I had a terrible time when Carrie came out. I was devastated and he didn't care. I'd shout at him, 'How can you not care?' He got furious with me. 'Don't tell me your reality,' he'd yell back. It definitely affected our relationship." Elise now realizes that Jim's reaction made sense in light of his experiences. He worked with a lot of LGBT people and the fact that his daughter was a lesbian truly did not bother him in the same way as it did her.

If you and your spouse are at very different points, here's what you need to do:

• Assure your child that she is not the cause of the fighting but that the problem is one parent's inability to deal with the situation or the fact that you and your spouse have very different reactions. Remind her you have a process to go through, too.

• If the anxiety in the house has escalated to screaming and fighting, set aside a time to talk when you're both calm and when the children are out of the house.

• Work with your spouse to keep the lines of communication open. You might begin by saying, "I know we have very different reactions to Jon's coming out. We need to talk about what's going on for each of us." Then lay out where you are and ask him to do the same.

• Continue to check in with each other from time to time, so you don't grow apart. It's easy to avoid this topic since it's so painful, but silence can undermine a marriage.

• Try to let go and let your spouse come to terms in his own way and in his own time, rather than put your reaction and timetable on him.

ACCEPTANCE AND BEYOND

When many parents first learn that their child is LGBT, they are overwhelmed by a huge range of negative emotions: guilt, shame, embarrassment, sadness. The fact that they love their child gets lost in a sea of other emotions and they lose sight of what's really important: understanding, loving and supporting their child. Ultimately, negative attitudes can lead to the child's alienation.

Parents find that when they can begin to get back in touch with their love for their child and realize the pain she is experiencing, that paves the way for true acceptance.

The turning point in Cher and Chastity's relationship came when Cher realized that she did not want to lose her daughter. In Chastity's memoir, Cher recalls, "I had to decide what to do with this information—do I turn my back, or go, 'Fine, I have to understand this. This is part of who she is and she's my child and I don't want to give up my relationship with her, and so I have do to this.'? There had been this barrier between us for such a long time, for years and years and years, part of me wanted, needed for it to disappear."

Keeping secrets is stressful and creates strain and generally leads to some kind of change in a child's demeanor or behavior and in others' reactions to her. Once those secrets are finally broken, there's a huge range of emotions. For some people it will be a relief and a delight to finally deal with the truth and for others, it may be hard at first to accept the news. But by breaking the silence and getting the issue out on the table, you are on the path to things getting better—even if the first wave of reactions is negative. The real threat is not naming the problem, because you can't deal with a problem if it is not acknowledged.

Here are four ways that have produced turning points for other parents:

1. ATTENDING PFLAG MEETINGS. This was a significant juncture for Anne. "I couldn't get enough of talking to people who understood and had gone through the same thing," she recalls. Many, many parents feel this way.

   On the other hand, if you and your spouse are at different stages of acceptance, you may be ready to go to a PFLAG meeting and your husband is not. You want to be proactive and supportive of your child but may end up feeling caught between your child and your husband. There is no easy solution to this situation. It is important that you get the support you need at PFLAG. Hopefully, with time, your husband will join you.

2. TALKING TO YOUR CLERGY. Be sure to take into consideration his or her views and your relationship with him or her. Terri, a practicing Catholic, felt she had to talk to her priest although she dreaded the meeting for weeks. "What should I do, Father?" she pleaded with the priest. She will never forget his answer. She recalls, "He said, 'You don't have to do anything. All you have to do is love him.' It was incredible. I thought he'd condemn me. I was floating. After that, things fell into place for me."

3. READING ABOUT LGBTQ ISSUES. This takes the focus off you and your personal struggles. When you become more knowledgeable about homosexuality, it may lessen your guilt and shame. Learning about the discrimination and homophobia your child may experience can help you focus on your child and make you more sensitive to her needs.

4. GAINING STRENGTH FROM YOUR CHILD. When Nikki told her mother that she was dating a woman, her mother tried to minimize it, telling her it was just a phase and would be over soon. Nikki told her she thought it was real. She recalls, "It was very disheartening because I did not feel affirmed at all. So I took that to mean, don't bring it up again, or bring it up when you have better news—like there's a boy involved." She continued to date this woman for a year and a half; neither she nor her mother ever mentioned it again.

Today, five years later, Nikki is involved with another woman and her mother adores her. What brought her mother around? Nikki reflects, "I stuck to my guns about who I am. The longevity of our relationship helps too—we've been together almost two years. I think it's a lot of work on the child's part to really stand strong in who you are and just being really tough about it. Saying 'This is someone who is really important in my life' and 'If you want to be in my life, then you need to accept this person.' Not just, can you sit in the same room with her, but can you embrace my lifestyle? I've just made a decision that unless you accept me with open arms, I really don't want to be around you."

With true acceptance, a degree of comfort exists so that your child's orientation becomes integrated into the family life and not the major focus of concern. A teenage girl remarked about the casualness with which her family now talks about her girlfriends, "My father and I never had a 'Dad, I'm gay' kind of discussion but I'll say, 'Oh, I want a girlfriend.' And I'll talk about my girlfriends and stuff. I can talk pretty openly with him." This degree of openness came about because she felt accepted and loved for who she is. She felt no shame talking about her girlfriends.

Oftentimes, just a small but very genuine comment can

mean a lot to your child and show her that your acceptance is heartfelt. One young woman recalls, "There was one sweet thing my mom said once, probably a year or so after I came out. My mom was scratching my head—a little affection thing she does when we watch TV or whatever. I made some obnoxious comment like, 'Oh, who's going to do this when you're dead?' She paused and said, 'Oh, your husband or life partner.' It was such a sweet little afterthought. Now we can tell lesbian jokes and they're funny."

If your daughter has a girlfriend (or your son, a boyfriend), here are several ways you can signal to her that you accept that fact:

- Ask how her girlfriend is doing or inquire about the relationship.
- Say, "Let's all go out to dinner" or make a point of saying, "I really like so-and-so."
- Treat their relationship with the same respect and rules that you use for your straight children. If you don't let your son sleep in the same bedroom with his girlfriend, tell your daughter's girlfriend, "You'll have to sleep in the other room," too. (You can break that rule once you've thrown them a huge commitment ceremony and paid for the catering, flowers, and other expenses!)

SIBLINGS' PROCESS

A child's coming out affects the entire nuclear and extended family—not just the person who comes out. As a parent, you have to help siblings go through their own "coming out" process. How siblings cope with the process is the result of two major factors:

1. Their relationship with the sib who's coming out. Generally, the stronger the relationship between the siblings, the more likely the coming out process will go
well. If they already have a strong relationship, one of
two things can happen. The first is that they may have
already confided in the sibling and found a strong sense
of support there. A second is that coming out may cause
a hiccup in the relationship. This isn't necessarily permanent: later on, the fact that they have weathered this
can draw them closer.

   If there's already a negative relationship, this will
make coming out harder. In one family I counseled, the
middle child was the one who came out. The older child
went to a military school, is religious, and never liked his
artsy little brother. His brother's coming out felt like one
more reason to dislike and resent his younger sib. But
disaster is not inevitable. In some cases where a negative
relationship between siblings has existed, "coming out"
may remove an unspoken barrier to a more positive relationship and can be an opportunity for the siblings to
grow closer.

   Parents play a crucial role in whether the coming out
process strengthens or weakens family bonds. It is critical that parents emphasize that membership in the family is not conditional. You can say to the son who is
having a hard time accepting his younger brother coming out, "You are entitled to your opinion but your
brother is still your brother and he is still our son, and
that's not negotiable." This message needs to be repeated like a broken record.

   Your LGBT child may fear that he'll be ejected from
the family. Therefore, as a parent, you need to affirm
that the family integrity won't crack. We can also be
hopeful that the brother's coming out will create new av-

enues of discussion and eventually lead to more closeness. If that happens between you and your LGBT
child, it has a good chance it can happen between your
LGBT child and his siblings.

2. The age of the sibling and the birth order. When sibs are
younger than your LGBT child, they may not have the
cognitive ability or vocabulary to understand what the
news means. You need to find age appropriate ways to
explain issues to a five year old, for example. Younger
children don't necessarily understand what people "do
in bed" but they do understand the concepts of love,
marriage, and family. You can explain that your LGBT
child may as an adult form a family with people of the
same sex, instead of the opposite sex.

The way you handle the coming out process also
shows the younger sibling how his parents deal with conflict. If you handle this badly, the younger sibs will get the
message: don't bring anything difficult to mom and dad.

A younger sib may also be confused by what's going
on and wonder, will this happen to me? This child needs
reassurance that each child is different and unique and
just because his older brother is gay, it doesn't mean that
he will be.

If the child who is coming out is younger than his siblings,
two dynamics are common:

1. Younger children often value the opinions and respect of
their older siblings and may fear that they'll lose that status by coming out. They need reassurance that nothing
has changed in the family dynamics and they are still
loved as much as before they came out. Help older sibs
remember how vulnerable they felt when they were your
LGBT child's age.

2. The coming out process inevitably focuses the family's
attention on the LGBT child. For older siblings, who

may feel that the younger children already gets special attention and privileges, this may cause some resentment and anger. It is important to discuss openly with siblings (of any age) that when a family member faces a special challenge, everyone needs to "go the extra mile" to support him.

To help you understand what your other children are going through, we've listed some of the common feelings siblings experience when their brother or sister comes out. They include:

Confusion. Younger sibs may not understand what's going on while older sibs have a wide range of reactions. Some may feel betrayed, thinking, "I thought I knew you. We came from the same family. How did this happen?" For others, learning they have a LGBT sibling is no big deal. They may have suspected for years. Still others will be shocked. Try to figure out where your child is along the confusion spectrum and what he needs. Most need information and guidance.

Anxiety—both for themselves and for their sibling's safety. Some siblings wonder whether they are going to lose their status in their peer group because they have an LGBT sib. They worry that they might be perceived as LGBT, too, and that they will be picked on. Many are also very concerned that their sibling will be harassed. You need to initiate an honest discussion about bigotry and what you're going to do to make them safe. Again, both siblings and LGBT youth need to hear the same message: that you're going to stick by them and help keep them safe.

Resentment often results for two reasons:

1. They resent the repercussions of their sibling's coming out. They may be angry that their own social status has been jeopardized. Or if their sibling's coming out in-

volves loss or disruption of the family, jeopardizes membership in a religious institution, or causes a rift with a family member, the non-LGBT sibling may feel a sense of loss. Before, everything was fine. Now, they may blame their LGBT sibling for this.

2. They resent that their sib is getting all the attention. Maybe they felt that the child who came out was already spoiled and their parent's favorite. Coming out makes the parents focus even more on this child and makes the sib feel left out and not as special.

Here are four key things for you to do if you sense resentment:

1. Listen to where the sibs are on the confusion spectrum. Determine the source of their anxiety and their resentment, if that's what they're feeling. Address it directly with them, giving them the space to express it. Then try to help them understand their sibling's perspective, and ask them how they would want to be treated if they were in that situation. Once their feelings are validated and their perspective is broadened, many will be more willing to be an ally for their sibling.

2. Continue to reemphasize that the family is one unit, that membership is equal for everyone and is not conditional.

3. Recognize that the coming out process will take time and energy—for everyone. Don't become so preoccupied with your LGBT child that you ignore the other children. Explain to them why it is taking up so much time and energy, perhaps by reminding them of a time when they needed extra time and energy and you and/or their siblings provided it. And remind them: this won't last forever. Someday things will go "back to normal."

4. Don't isolate younger sibs. Include them in the process, regardless of their age. Too many parents try to "protect" younger siblings, not understanding their need to understand what's going on, too, and to be able to express their feelings about it. They need the solidity of the family affirmed and they need to feel that they aren't on the sidelines or suffering consequences because of their sib's decision to come out.

BROADENING YOUR ACCEPTANCE: TELLING OTHERS

Deciding whom to tell, when to tell them and how to do it should be a joint decision, driven largely by your child. Respect where your child is in her process and also take into consideration where you are in yours. Coming out to family and friends should be done intentionally, so that you and your child negotiate it together.

While your child may be more eager to tell others because she may be a step or two ahead of you, you may have more sensitivity to family issues and sentiments. Families get into trouble when they haven't thought this out or when someone suddenly blurts out at the Thanksgiving table, "Tommy has a boyfriend."

As you're thinking about whom to tell when, and how you're going to break the news, keep in mind certain points:

- Don't make assumptions, particularly about older people. They are not all bigoted. Many of them may know a lot more about LGBT people than you think and have been around a long time and have seen it all.
- Do assume that people will be accepting and supportive. Give them the benefit of the doubt.

- Do assume that people start from a base line of loving their family members, and that you can work with them to help them understand someone who is different from them.
- Understand that your relatives also have to go through a process. Be prepared to give them the time, space and support they need as they move through it.

The same two factors that shaped your process in dealing with your child's coming out will determine how your relatives handle the news. Think them through again as you decide whom you tell and gauge their potential reaction:

1. What is their degree of awareness on homosexual issues?

   If you are unsure of how your relatives feel about LGBTQ issues, send out a trial balloon. You might say, "They just started a gay-straight alliance at Josh's school. I think it's great." Tell them about it and see how the relatives respond.

2. What is their relationship with your child?

   Those who are already close often value the relationship enough to do what it takes to keep it intact. Evaluate their relationship by considering:
   - how close family members are to your child
   - how often they see her
   - the nature of their relationship

Then, consider their relationship in light of their awareness of LGBT issues. Gertie explains how she and her son, Adam, decided whom to tell in their family. "Adam told his two cousins, now seventeen and sixteen, that he was gay and my sister knows but her husband doesn't. I didn't tell him because he loves Adam and I don't want him to turn against Adam. But truth be told, he's a bigot. I'm not ashamed of Adam, but I don't want people to hurt him, and people who I think can't handle it, I won't tell. I told his cousins, 'Don't tell your father because this is Adam's thing and Adam is the one who should be able to decide whom to tell.' They know what their dad is really like."

Gertie's husband has three sisters and only one knows. "The other two are real religious fanatics," she says. "They have tunnel vision. They would still love Adam [if they knew], but they'd be on the phone every minute trying to change him and he doesn't need that aggravation. Therefore, we didn't tell them."

Another factor is important in deciding whom to tell: The amount of psychic energy you expend by *not* telling close family and friends. One father recalls the emotional toll of keeping his son's secret. "I also began to realize that being closeted . . . required emotional and psychic energy that interfered with close personal relationships. Before I spent an evening with friends, I'd have to recall exactly what I'd told them on previous occasions. During the time we were together I kept a diversionary discussion topic ready at a moment's notice to interject into the conversation if necessary. On the way home I wondered if what I'd said was consistent with our previous times together. I was beginning to feel paranoid about keeping all these things straight in my mind. There were times I felt a scorecard for each family and friend was the only solution."

Eventually this father talked to his son about how the burden of silence was affecting him. His son agreed that his father could come out to close friends, but that coming out to family would be done by the son at times and methods of his choosing.

Before you come out to others, talk to other parents of LGBTQ teens. You will find them at a local PFLAG meeting. Ask them some of the following questions:

- how they came out to others
- whom they told first

- what kind of responses they got
- what other advice they have for taking this big step.

Decide with your child whom you are going to tell and how by following these five steps:

1. Sit down together at a time when neither of you is rushed and go through the list of close family members. Begin with your parents or siblings. For example, you might say, "What about Aunt Annie?"
2. Evaluate your child's relationship with her as well as your own by answering the following questions:
   - How often does your daughter see her?
   - What is the nature of their relationship?
   - Would you feel dishonest not sharing something so important with your sister?
3. Consider whether she accepts diversity and her attitudes toward homosexuality, if you know them. Discuss together:
   - How accepting is she of people who are different?
   - What was her reaction when one of her children brought home a friend of a different race?
   - Do you have any evidence that she's homophobic?
4. Decide who will break the news:
   - you
   - your child
   - you and your child together.

   Let your child be the guide here and go with her preferences unless you strongly disagree. Evaluate who is more comfortable with the family member and who will have an opportunity to talk. Say you and your daughter agree that your sister should know, but your daughter only sees her a few times a year and you talk to her every week. In that case, it would make more sense for you to break the news on the phone.

5. Just do it.

What do you actually say? Here is a good example that shows the importance of timing, sensitivity and opening up the subject gradually. Liz, who is a lesbian, came out to grandmother about a year after she told her mother. Liz waited until her grandfather was taking a nap, and then said, 'Nana, there's something I want to tell you and it has to do with my personal life."

"You had a baby?"

"No, Nana."

"You almost had a baby?"

"No."

"You like girls more than you like boys."

"Yeah."

Her grandmother smiled and said, "Yeah."

Liz recalls, "It was very sweet." Her grandmother then went on in a matter-of-fact way to discuss with her whom they should and shouldn't tell in the family. This worked because of their unconditional love. No doubt, Liz's grandmother was flattered by her granddaughter's openness.

To sum up:

- Be clear about your motives for making the disclosure, and be prepared for whatever consequences (good or bad) it may bring.
- Choose a time to talk when you won't be interrupted.
- Pick a place that's private, so other people aren't coming in and out.
- Select a time when you're feeling strong emotionally and not upset, distracted or angry.

- Begin with a general statement, such as, "There's something I want to tell you" or "There's something I want to share with you of a personal nature."
- Then say something like, "Liz dates girls" or "Bill has a boyfriend." Many people find these statements easier to say than "My daughter is a lesbian" or "My son is gay."
- Apply the same listening skills you use with your child when you are discussing this with a family member.

FINDING SUPPORT FOR YOUR CHILD

To help your child feel good about herself and normalize her experience, encourage her to be around peers who are LGBT. Even if you are still struggling with your own issues, this is a way to support her.

There are four primary ways that youth build communities for themselves. They are:

LGBT youth support groups in schools. The most prominent of these groups are gay-straight alliances (GSAs), which are clubs started by students in high schools to support one another and to combat homophobia. There are now over 1,000 alliances in 47 states. To find out more about GSAs and similar clubs, go to our web site, www.glsen.org

Community-based support centers. These centers, such as The Attic in Philadelphia, are a wonderful resource for LGBTQ teens to meet other teens. The problem is, however, that they are mainly in big cities and if a child is underage, either not out to her parents or has unsupportive parents and must rely on them for transportation, she will have difficulty getting to one of these groups.

Informal support networks. These include drama clubs, softball teams and other organizations that are not LGBTQ on the surface, but for a variety of reasons may have a more LGBT-friendly atmosphere. Some groups are often targeted as being for people who are LGBTQ, so some teens purposely shun them to avoid being identified.

The Internet. Finding support online is very appealing to teens who are not out or who have unsupportive parents, because they find instant support, they don't have to travel, and they can remain anonymous. However, if you're like many parents, you're probably frightened by the prospect of your child surfing the net, alone in cyberspace, prey to malicious strangers with false identities. But the fact is: The Internet provides a safe haven for countless LGBTQ teenagers who are not out to their families or who do not have family support—provided it is used with the guidelines I'm about to give you.

The following example will show you the benefit of online relationships, so you can understand how your child might feel when she connects online with someone else who's LGBTQ. Michael, who lives in Georgia, didn't even admit to himself that he was gay until his senior year of high school. The first person he came out to was an online pen pal, Troy, who wrote to him because his profile mentioned that Bebe Neuwirth was one of his favorite performers; Troy loved her as well. Troy told him about his experience with guys; Michael admitted that he wasn't sure about his orientation, but thought he might be gay.

They wrote emails back and forth for months, Michael sharing concerns and doubts that he hadn't shared with a real live person. They then started instant messaging each other. Michael recalls, "We just supported each other through the whole process. He went to a performing arts high school in New York and I came from a small town in the South, so we had very different experiences. He felt fairly comfortable with the whole idea of being gay—more than I did—because he had been exposed to it much more."

Troy is the only person Michael has ever developed a relationship with online. With Troy's support, Michael got the courage to come out to his family. He and Troy still correspond and met last summer when Michael came up north; they had a lot of fun together. Sometimes Michael goes online to talk with younger guys who are having trouble coming out. "It makes me feel like I'm doing some good for someone," he said.

Michael is honest and well-meaning, but some adults, especially those posing as students, can have ulterior motives. Because of its anonymity, the Internet can create instant intimacy, but it can be a dangerous place for someone who feels isolated and vulnerable. If a child has no one to turn to or talk openly to in (real) life, online relationships can become overly important. An isolated, alienated child can be vulnerable to anyone who shows a little caring and understanding.

That said, however, I am not a big supporter of filtering software. Most youth are much more sophisticated technically than their parents and know how to outsmart the filtering system. In addition, much of the software is inconsistent and blocks out the good sites along with the bad.

When parents install such software, their children feel controlled, distrusted and that their parents are trying to separate them from their friends. This is hardly likely to strengthen a parent-child relationship, and it is also insensitive to the very real fact that many of these teens don't have real life communities: denying them Internet access may be denying them access to the only people they can "talk" to.

It is also very difficult to monitor the online habits of a teenager. Most parents work and many teens are left home alone weekday afternoons, evenings or weekends. This is where the trusting relationship you have developed with your teen will pay off. At a time when you are not rushed, sit down and have a discussion with your teen about the mixed blessings of the Internet. You can begin by saying something like, "The Internet is a wonderful thing. It gives you lots of access to information and people, and that's a good thing. Like most things in life, though, it's a mixed blessing. As people are in any setting, they may not be what they say they are."

Then, go on and say, "I respect you and trust you and expect you to do the right thing. Sometimes, you will do bad things and I won't catch you. If you do bad things and I do catch you, there will be consequences." More important, try to teach your child how to judge for herself when her actions might have negative consequences, as you will not always be around to make those kinds of judgments for her.

Make sure to include the following points in your discussion:

- Be skeptical about what you read online.
  Everything you see is not true. Anyone can post
  information and just because it's there does not
  mean it's correct.
- Don't necessarily believe what someone tells you.
  Many people disguise themselves by creating
  fictitious identities. Someone who says he's a
  teen could actually be a forty-five-year-old man.
- Try to keep some distance so you don't get too
  attached to one person. People can disappear
  online as fast as they surface.

Following your discussion about the dangers of the Internet, tell your teen that you want her to agree to certain rules for her safety. The best way to make rules that your child will abide by is to involve her in that process and make it a collaborative one: If she helps make the rules, she'll be more likely to follow them. From your perspective, some of the following might be ones you offer as possibilities. Write or type them on a sheet of paper and present them to your child.

I agree:

- I will use an alias at all times.
- I will never give out our last name, address, phone number or other personal information, such as my school name or athletic team. If someone asks where I live, I'll give a general answer, like South Florida or northern Illinois. I won't give the name of my city.
- I will not give out my password to anyone.
- If anything I see or do makes me feel uncomfortable, I will tell a parent.
- I won't offer any sexual details, no matter how "in need" the other party seems.
- I will not send anyone a photo of myself or my family
- I will not click on a page that says, "For over 18 years only." If I go there accidentally, I will leave.
- I will never meet someone in person whom I've met online, unless I have discussed it with you first and do so in a public place at a time you are aware of.

After you have discussed these and/or other rules, make a copy of the ones you agree on and ask your teen to sign the bottom of the page.

This is a discussion that you will need to have more than once. After the initial discussion, go back a month later and see how things are going. See where the problem areas are and whether your child is following the rules, or if you and she need to reconsider some of them. Most of all, keep the discussion going.

With your support, your child will go online safely. She won't go meet someone and fall into a harmful relationship out of desperation.

FINDING SUPPORT FOR YOURSELF

When you meet parents of other LGBTQ teenagers, you won't feel so isolated. You'll recognize that many other parents have gone through a similar process. You may find it helpful to talk with others who are at the same stage as you, as well as with those who have known for a while to see how they've coped. The primary organization for parents, PFLAG (www.pflag.org), has members from 80,000 households with 450 affiliates worldwide.

For one father, attending his first PFLAG meeting allowed him to begin opening his own closet door. He recalls, "For the first time in a year, I felt understood and accepted by others who had walked in my shoes. So, once a month I cautiously unlocked my closet door and went to a parents' meeting—only returning home a few hours later to barricade myself in for another four weeks."

Each month, he received support, information and most important, hope. He continues, "It was at those meetings that I began to replace a lifetime of misinformation with reliable facts about homosexuality. There, too, I met other parents who shared my feelings and experiences. Some of them seemed freer of the demons and fears that haunted me. They, in a sense, held out a vision of what was possible for me too. I vividly remember a parent saying, 'I'm proud of my daughter; she's a wonderful young woman. I wouldn't trade her for the world.' I, too, was proud of my child. But something held me back. Although I tried to analyze that hesitancy on numerous occasions, I never arrived at a satisfactory explanation."

Books are another important resource for parents. Check out the reading list at the back of this book for an extensive list of books that may be helpful to you. Some are personal accounts of parents of LGBTQ children, others offer guidelines and advice about what to expect at each stage of the process. Reading these books will give you support and information. The more you know, the more comfortable you'll feel with your child's orientation, the better you'll be able to support her, and the stronger your relationship will become.

WHERE DO WE GO FROM HERE?

Some parents, once they learn that their child is LGBTQ, never bring up the subject again. It is the elephant in the room that no one talks about. I would encourage you, however, to make the coming-out conversation the first of many. Even if you feel uncomfortable in the beginning, it is important to encourage these discussions because they help normalize your child's sexuality and your connection with her.

What do you actually talk about in subsequent conversations? Ritch Savin-Williams suggests, "Encourage the child to share his or her history of same-sex attractions, the ways in which sexual orientation has influenced the child's life, who else knows and how they have reacted, and future expectations the youth has about his or her life as a gay person."

The way to begin these discussions is to talk about yourself and your experiences. The reflections you've done in the early chapters have probably brought stories and experiences to mind. One night after dinner, you (the dad) might reminisce, "I remember when I was in second grade and little Susie Smith came in and she had blonde pigtails. I just thought she was the cutest thing. I didn't really realize that I was straight but there was something different about Susie that attracted me. I'm wondering if it's the same for people who are gay. Did you ever have a feeling like that?"

This helps your child see that you've grappled with these issues and are open to learning about her experiences. You can even say, "All I know is my own experiences. I would really like to learn about yours, because you probably have a different experience than mine and we grew up in different time periods. There are probably a lot of ways our experiences are the same and probably ways they are totally different. I would be really intrigued to find out what those are."

This type of conversation humanizes you. It reminds your child that you were once young too (which is easy for her to forget) and that you didn't always have all the answers either. That's reassuring to teens.

The fact that your child came out to you is a gift. It is a way to know your child better, more honestly and more completely. Handle it with care, and your family can grow in understanding, compassion and intimacy.

Chapter Six

THE TRANSGENDERED TEEN

"I WAS BORN in a female body and my parents expected a girl and thought they had a girl and treated me like a girl. But it didn't work. That wasn't who I was," recalls Jamison, a transsexual man.

"I was an extremely androgynous child. I grew up in the fifties and sixties and had to wear a dress to school. There was no wearing jeans or pants of any kind. So I felt cross-dressed every single day. I was really miserable and yet I had no way to express any kind of resistance to this because of my female body. I was just expected to wear this clothing, which gave messages to other people about who I was."

"Even when I was wearing a dress, people couldn't tell what sex I was," Jamison continues. "They were constantly asking me: 'Are you a boy or a girl?' I remember clearly from the time I was six or seven years old, all the way through college when of course I stopped wearing dresses, people still asked me whether I was a boy or a girl. That's because my gender was always masculine. So when I changed my sex, I didn't change my gender."

Jamison represents an increasingly visible population that has special needs and concerns: transgendered individuals. Transgender is an umbrella term covering all people whose gender identity and expression do not conform to what is expected of them based on their biological sex and who live substantial portions of their lives as other than their birth sex. It includes "mannish" women, cross-dressers, transsexuals who have undergone gender reassignment surgery, like Jamison, and "gender benders," like David Bowie, Boy George and k. d. lang, who merge the characteristics of both sexes.

Trans individuals share in common the belief that their biological sex and attributes don't match how they feel inside. For example, a girl may be born with female biological characteristics but dress like a boy, cut her hair short and act very masculine. The other students ridicule her and call her a dyke, even though she may not be a lesbian.

The literal visibility of their difference marks them for persecution in ways that LGB youth, who can sometimes more easily pass, do not always face. The profound ignorance of society means that they are even less likely to find support than their LGB peers. And the discomfort of many within the LGB movement with the "T" means that even the logical community for transgendered people is not always an affirming place.

Transgendered youth face many of the same issues that LGB youth face, but they also face additional challenges unique to them. Trans teenagers can be in terrible pain, as the following excerpt from a trans teen's journal illustrates: "Fuck being trans . . . It is such a fucking pain in the ass to try and be my fucking self. Why can't people just leave me alone?? I don't want to draw attention to myself . . . I just want to be. I hate this. I hate this passionately. Sometimes it sucks to actually be passable as a boy. Everyone who knows you as a girl thinks that you are ugly, because you don't fit into the mold of who they think you should be . . . God damn it, I am hurting right now."

These teens may grow up with a deep sense of shame and feel as though they can't express themselves authentically with the body they've been given. Many people just can't stand it when girls don't "act like girls" and boys don't "act like boys." Consequently, transgendered people can be harassed and discriminated against even more than gay men and lesbians, because they are so visible and their image often clashes with typical gender stereotypes.

As the parent of a trans teen, you have a particularly challenging task: to accept your child for who he is and to give him the support he so desperately needs. In this chapter, we'll cover what you need to know to do that. I'll explain what it means to be transgendered, how to tell whether your child is LGB or transgendered, how to understand what your child is experiencing in school and other areas of society and how to cope with issues specific to transgendered teens, such as changing their name, having reassignment surgery and handling harassment.

Lastly, I'll suggest ways to find support for yourself and your child.

WHAT DOES TRANSGENDERED MEAN?

In defining transgender, it's helpful to think about the difference between sex and gender. We often use these terms interchangeably but they are not the same. Many people think they are because their own gender and sex are in alignment. In fact, there are great variations in masculine and feminine qualities with respect to male and female bodies.

Here are the key definitions you need to know:

• Sex is how society defines us based on the appearance of biological characteristics, such as reproductive organs, when a baby is born. When we talk about sex, we use the words female and male.

• Gender is about the spirit inside a given body, the personality, behavior, feelings that reinforce the maleness or femaleness of the body, regardless of the body's sex. When we talk about gender, we use the words feminine and masculine.

• Gender expression is how we externally communicate our gender, through behaviors or modes of dress—whatever you engage in that has gender connotations. Many LGB and straight people experience and express their gender in ways consistent with what society expects based on their biological sex. Trans people can't or don't.

• Gender identity is the innermost sense of self: how you perceive yourself and how you want others to perceive you.

We talked in Chapter 2 about how LGB youth often stay closeted by presenting themselves as straight and their peers often think they're straight. Trans teens, too, can bury their feelings behind "proper" behavior, trying to fit in, but eventually they will have to express the frustration they feel because their gender and their bodies don't "line up" the way most people's do.

Lori, for example, was an attractive girl from a small farming community in Oregon where girls were expected to be strong and athletic. Everyone thought her energy and liveliness were endearing qualities. She kept her blond hair short because she was on the high school swim team, and when she earned a varsity letter, she ordered the boy's sweater. Some kids teased her, even though the boy's sweater looked great on her. No one knew how she really felt; but to her, that varsity letter meant she had become one of the boys, because inside she knew she was a boy, no matter what anyone else thought. She had reassignment surgery (what used to be called a sex change operation) in her mid-twenties, and is a man today with a wife and two sons.

In many cases, transgendered youth are quite visible because they are unable to hide or mask their gender difference. Adolescence can be hell for them, because they feel as if they are developing the adult body of the "wrong" sex and it's totally inconsistent with their own inner expression or identity. While most teenage boys can't wait to have enough facial hair to shave, a biologically male, transgendered boy might find facial hair repulsive. In the same way, a biologically female, transgendered girl would feel betrayed by her body when she begins to menstruate and develop breasts. She was hoping to become more masculine as she got older.

Hard as it may be for you to understand, the fact is: What your child is feeling inside is true and real for him, despite society's expectations or his biological sex, or what his body "tells him" based on what we know about biology.

A national survey of 1000 parents of five- to eighteen-year-olds conducted from July 31 to August 7, 2001 found the following:

- By a slim margin, more parents agree that schools should teach tolerance and respect for students who express their gender identity in nontraditional ways than agree that schools should encourage boys and girls to act traditionally.
- Parents who are most likely to agree that schools should teach respect for students with nontraditional gender identities include people with gay family members or close friends, and those who believe homosexuality is innate and not a moral issue. Secular parents, unmarried moms and suburban moms are also more willing than parents in general to express this view.

IS MY CHILD LGB OR TRANSGENDERED? OR BOTH? OR NEITHER?

Many people automatically assume that transgendered teens are LGB. That is not necessarily true. They can be LGB or straight, but because they are so often ostracized by the straight community, they sometimes find more acceptance with LGB people, but that does not necessarily mean that they are LGB.

While similarities can exist in how LGB and trans teens

appear to the world, there is a huge difference between them. The defining issue for LGB people is sexual orientation: whom they are attracted to. That is not true for transgendered people. Their defining issue is their gender identity: how they perceive themselves and how others perceive them, not their sexual orientation.

As a parent, you may be wondering how to tell whether your child is LGB or transgender. There are no hard and fast rules. In the past, some saw certain styles of clothes as a giveaway, but this is no longer true because there is so much experimentation with clothes today. Of course, clothing styles and their relationship to gender have always evolved: Think of how "proper young ladies" of the fifties never wore slacks, because they were considered "unladylike," whereas our Founding Fathers wore wigs, which were considered "masculine" then.

The following clues may signal that your child is transgendered but they can also be signs of other things, so evaluate them carefully in light of everything else that you know about your child and with what you observe about him:

1. Pronounced cross-dressing

   For girls—By 1950s standards virtually all women today "cross-dress." But a trans girl might take such dress to the extreme by dressing in ways that are exaggeratedly masculine. She might wear a jacket and tie or a tuxedo. She may refuse to wear a skirt under any circumstances.

   Trans girls may try to hide their breasts by walking hunch shouldered, covering them with layers of clothing or wearing oversized, loose tops. Some girls even bind their breasts with tape. Keep in mind, though, that there may be other reasons why young girls hide their secondary sex characteristics. For example, some studies have shown this can also be a sign that a girl has been sexually abused or sexually harassed. The important thing to remember is that when you see these signs, they are telling you that something is going on: Pay attention to it.

For boys—When I was in high school, wearing an earring was definitely "gender deviant" for boys and would get any boy who did so labeled "gay." Today, virtually every high school football player seems to sport an earring, so notions of masculine dress have clearly changed in a very short time. Today boys get their ears pierced, paint their fingernails and some wear skirts occasionally. But there are still "invisible" lines around gender for boys, and habitually dressing in "female" clothes earns swift wrath from peers. Consequently boys tend to be "closet" cross-dressers, dressing up at home and not in public.

2. An expressed aversion to gender-stereotyped activities but when asked why your son prefers cooking, for example, to baseball, he cannot give you a reason. This may also be true of LGB youth, so this clue alone would not be telling.

3. Wanting to change his given name and either choosing an androgynous name or a name of the other sex.

Jamison recalls, "I changed my name to Chip and then I was Thor, god of thunder. But when I was in junior high I was the only girl in wood shop, so the guys named me Bill. One day someone called my home and asked for Bill and my mother said, 'There is no one here by that name.' I said, 'What name, mom?' And she goes, 'Bill' and I said, 'Oh, it's for me.'"

He continues, "My mother seemed annoyed, but she let me take the call. It was one of my classmates. I think my parents (my mother in particular) felt my behavior was just a stage that I would outgrow any minute, and the sooner the better."

4. Something different about your child. It's very hard to pinpoint, but some parents say, "I've known that my son was a girl from the time that he was three years old. He just walked differently, he just reacted to things differently. He wasn't like other male children in our family."

Because we have such rigid gender standards in this country, anyone who bends the roles and rules will stand out. Gender differences may show up at a young age for both boys and girls.

Our society is so protective of masculinity that any deviation in a young boy is addressed swiftly and often harshly very early on. Thus boys are punished more aggressively and earlier than girls are for gender-variant behavior. Boys learn very quickly to hide or suppress their feelings. They tend to blame themselves and hold the belief that something is horribly wrong with them.

Girls, on the other hand, seem to have a certain leeway for "tomboy" behavior that may not be extended to boys. They may not get aggressive gender conforming messages until they are older and psychologically stronger and more able to differentiate their own feelings from those of people around them.

But sooner or later all youth, regardless of biology, have to cope with the demands of a society that has clear expectations around gender.

ADDRESSING THE SIGNS

If your child has some of the tendencies we discussed above, don't ignore them or belittle them. Don't assume that when your daughter gets into high school, for example, and meets boys, she's going to change and want to wear makeup and skirts. Society tells you it's going to pass and you may hope it will, and it may, but it may not. Allow your child to develop naturally without trying to change or evaluate him.

If you notice any of the signs above, note them and let your child respond. For example, if you find a pair of high heels in your son's closet when you're cleaning, note your observation by saying something like, "I found a pair of high heels in your closet when I was putting away your laundry today. I'm wondering what they were doing there." Let your son take it from there. Try to keep an open mind and listen to what he has to say. Brush up on the communication skills we discussed in the first chapter, so he will feel more comfortable telling you what's really going on.

Keep in mind that your child may not be ready to respond yet because he isn't comfortable talking about it with you, so keep your questions open-ended and non-threatening, and let your child respond in the time frame that works for him.

Part of you may not want to have this discussion at all, hoping that if you don't talk about it, it will go away. But it won't. Discussing it now rather than later could save your son years of unhappiness, because he will not have to hide and sneak, but can be open about his preferences.

ACCEPTING YOUR TRANSGENDERED TEEN

The most common reaction on learning that a child is transgendered is denial. The parent withdraws, doesn't want to have contact with anyone, refuses to admit his or her child might have any issues and is absolutely unwilling to deal with it. Parents in denial make comments like the following:

"She's just a late bloomer."

"There's nothing wrong with my child."

"It's just a phase. He'll outgrow it."

This can cause tremendous stress for your child. The more resistance and rigidity you express, the more that is going to polarize your relationship with him, which could lead to increased fighting, distancing and hostility.

On the other hand, your reaction is perfectly understandable. It is not surprising that you are upset about having a trans child, considering the way society trained you. You've been raised in a culture that told you that because your child has certain physical characteristics, you can expect certain things to happen in his life. No one equipped you to know what to do. So if you feel confused or upset, that's okay. There has been nothing in our society to date or probably in your life that would have equipped you to be anything except confused and upset.

In the last chapter, we discussed the parent's process of accepting her LGB child. That same process applies here. However, the following two issues are more pronounced in parents of trans teens:

1. A lot of parents of trans teens feel their own sense of masculinity or femininity threatened. While some parents of LGB youth feel this as well, parents of trans youth tend to have a stronger reaction in this area.

   It's particularly hard for the parent of the same biological gender as the child. Fathers are typically threatened by a transgendered son and mothers, by a trans daughter. This is because parents tend to see the behavior of their children as validating or diminishing their own life choices, including those around gender expression.

   That is, a mother feels her life choices are justified when her daughter marries and has a family, as she did. On the other hand, when her daughter is transgendered or even a lesbian, a mother can interpret her daughter's lifestyle as a rejection of her own. Of course, this is not true. Being transgendered or a lesbian is not a choice and is not about the mother. It's about your child living an authentic life.

   If you are struggling with this issue, here's what can help:

- Try to separate your choices from those of your child. You are two different people.
- Try to give your child the space to be authentic—even if you think the results "reflect badly" on you. In truth, the only "bad reflection" on a parent is when a parent has put her own agenda ahead of her child's real needs. Go back to Chapter 1 and do the self-reflection exercises again if you need to.
- Remember that you can't force your child to be someone he's not—not without exacting a terrifying price, so do your best to let go and move toward acceptance.

2. Not only can trans children push your buttons about gender and other issues, but they create an enormous amount of fear, even for parents who desperately want their child to act the way they know is true for them. That is understandable. But for now, I'm asking you to put that aside, if you can, (I'll tell you how to deal with that later) and concentrate on how you can accept your child in the fullest sense of the word.

WORKING THROUGH YOUR OWN FEELINGS

It will take time for you to resolve your own issues. Give yourself that time and be patient with yourself. As we discussed in the last chapter, however, it's important that you begin that process by finding a place and means to resolve your feelings. Parents of trans teens often feel more isolated than parents of LGB teens, because transgenderism is not talked about a lot. Many otherwise-accepting people think of transgendered people as "perverted" or mentally ill in ways that LGB people are not.

To come to terms with your own issues, take time to reflect on the following areas:

• The fact that you have a transgendered child is not a reflection of your parenting, any more than having an LGB child is. You may be embarrassed or ashamed of the way your child looks or dresses, but his appearance is not about you. It's how he expresses who he really is.

• Try to let go of worrying about what other people think. Most people know very little about transgender issues, so they may have ignorant or insensitive reactions. Stay focused on what's most important: your child's well-being and self-esteem.

• Be patient with yourself. Give yourself time to process your feelings and realize that your process is unique. You may need to rethink your own attitudes toward gender, where they came from and why you have them.

• Learn as much as you can about transgender issues. The bibliography at the back of this book suggests several good texts. There are also videos and web sites that can be helpful to you.

• Try to step out of the traditional gender box. As you go about your business, notice others who dress in unconventional ways but who lead productive lives. If someone dresses in a way that you think is inappropriate for his or her gender, it's probably because you have some discomfort with it. Try to think about why that upsets you so much.

While you are reflecting on the issues above, take the following actions:

• Try to find a group of transgender people in your area, so you can gain some firsthand experience. You may have to be persistent: Transgender people can be shy, and a little wary of contact with non-transgendered parents. Many of them remember their own struggles with unforgiving parents and may be fearful of being blamed all over again. When you meet them, try to see beyond appearance and get to know them as individuals.

Here are three ways to find transgender groups:

1. Through a local LGBT center in your community.

2. Through a listing in LGBT community newspapers, even though many transgender groups have no LGB members (remember, it's not about sex. It's about gender).

3. Through the International Foundation for Gender Education (IFGE). IFGE maintains a very comprehensive listing of transgender community groups across the United States. A contact with one group close to your area can lead to others that are not listed in IFGE. Even if the group you first contact is composed primarily of older male-to-female people and you are looking for support for a female-to-male teen, someone in the group will usually know how to get in touch with some FTMs or younger people. Contact information is in the Resources section at the back of this book.

   If there are no such groups in your area, web sites, chat rooms, and list serves on the Internet provide alternative way of connecting.

• Go to a PFLAG meeting. Meet parents of other trans teens so you can share stories and learn about how they came to accept their child. PFLAG has a transgender special outreach network that can put you in touch with other parents if you are not able to find them in your local chapter. They also publish a work called "Our Trans Children" that can give you background information and advice.

• Go to your child's school and look at the wide variety of dress, hairstyle and clothing that teenagers wear today. Most teens are not dressed in khaki pants and button-down shirts. Your child might not be as "different" as you think after all.

If you've done all these things and still feel stuck or can't let go of your guilt, anger or sadness, think about getting counseling for yourself. Later in the chapter, I'll discuss how to find a good gender therapist.

SPECIAL ISSUES FOR TRANS TEENS

If you have a transgendered child, you may face some unique challenges. Below, I have listed some common problems and suggested ways for you to handle them.

My child wants to dress to the extreme as the other gender and I'm worried that he'll be harassed at school.

This fear is very real: Trans teens are 50 percent more likely to experience harassment at school than the general LGB population. Listen to the voice of a fifteen-year-old girl who explains some of the difficulties she experienced at school: "So many times I have been perceived as male—whether it's my clothes, my hair, my body composition or a combination of those, I don't know. People take things for granted—like being able to go into a public restroom and not be stared or screamed at. I hate going to the bathroom at school, 'cause every time I do, I catch someone off guard, and I can see that look of 'oh my God, there's a boy in the girls' bathroom' but then it fades.

"I remember one incident where this girl ran down the hall yelling that I was going into the wrong bathroom. I ignored her and proceeded to enter. She proceeded to follow me into the bathroom just to inform me that I was in the wrong place. She realized I was, in fact, a woman, called me a 'dyke,' and then left. Sure, I wear the pants, but that's no excuse or justification. . . . I get such strange looks that they have me convinced that I am, in fact, in the wrong place, that I am the one who doesn't belong."

To help your child avoid situations like this, you need to have serious conversations at home with him about the varying degrees to which he puts himself at risk and makes choices about how he shows the identity he feels inside. You might say, "Look, I know it's really hard for you not to fully express yourself in the clothes you wear, but if you wear that shirt/skirt/pants, you have a good chance of getting teased/bullied/beat up. I want you to be yourself, but we have to be realistic. I also want you to be safe."

Continue the discussion focusing on the following questions:

- How are kids on the bus/at school reacting to this?
- How does that make you feel?
- Have you thought about other reactions (including violence) people might have?
- Do you have a plan for dealing with these consequences?
- How does the possibility/reality of getting treated this way make you feel?

The key here is to make sure your child has thought through the consequences of his actions, and can make a thoughtful and well-reasoned decision about them. If your child is completely rational about his explanation and really wants to continue to do this, despite the possible negative consequences, then you might say, "Well, I want you to be safe. What can we do to increase your safety? Maybe I'll drive you to school. Or I'll go and talk with the bus driver or the school administrators." See how he reacts to those suggestions.

It's always difficult to strike the appropriate balance between being rightfully vigilant about your child's safety and being overprotective in a way that feels stifling. The real litmus test is when something puts your child at actual (not perceived, not projected, not anticipated) risk of harm, though this may be difficult to discern. If events unfold in such a way that you are truly worried for his safety, then follow these four steps:

1. If there is no safe place in the community for your child to cross-dress—or even if there is—make your home a safe haven. This is a particularly difficult issue for parents of boys who want to wear dresses. But in considering this, take into account these comments from teenage boys about how cross dressing consoled them when so much of their life was torturous.

   "I was sixteen when I started cross-dressing. I'd just reached mom's height, and she had a couple of wigs back then. So I'd wait until everyone was gone—I'd make excuses to be home alone—and then dress up and put on a wig. Then I'd just sit around and read. It was not stimulating, but it made me feel wonderful in so many ways. There was an overwhelming sense of everything finally being right. I remember being dizzy with exultation. In fact, I was always happy when I cross-dressed."

   Another young man said, "in my teens, after finding no outlet for communication and emotional discussion among my family or any male friends, I began to cross-dress whenever I had the chance. This gave me an immediate sense of comfort and satisfaction that seemed to help hold me over until the next time."

2. Say to him, "I know this feels authentic to you and I know this is the right way for you to act, but it's just not safe for you to do, so I cannot let you go to school dressed like that. I fear for your safety." Continue to repeat that message.

   You can also add, "I'm really sorry that you're in an unsafe environment. We're going to do everything we can about it. It's unfair to you and we're going to fight to make it fair. But until it is fair, we need to be realistic."

3. Again stress that you will try to change the circumstances, but in the meantime, he may want to modify the way he dresses. In Chapter 9 we will discuss how to advocate for your teen at school. Skip ahead to that chapter if you feel it would be helpful to you now.

4. Offer an alternative. Tell him, "Since you can't express yourself in a way that feels comfortable on the bus/at school, we'll find some place where you can, like the local community center, so there will be a time and place where you know you can be yourself, but this (the school setting) isn't it." Then, contact the school guidance counselor or local PFLAG chapter to find such places.

My son wants to wear a dress for Thanksgiving dinner and grandma is coming over and she doesn't know that he cross-dresses.

There are several ways you can handle this, but because people's personalities are so different, what might work in one family might not work in another. However you handle it, ultimately you need to make it clear that the needs of your child come first. It's devastating for a child to hear that you are more worried about what your own mother's going to think than how your child is going to feel. You're old enough to theoretically no longer need your parent's approval to feel secure; your child isn't.

I recommend that you involve your child in the decision. But if you do this, your child must know that you are not trying to push him into a particular answer and that you are prepared to genuinely support whichever answer he gives. Say just that to your child, to open the discussion.

Then tell him, "Look, you know grandma has certain prejudices. If it is essential to you to dress this way, I'm willing to call her and tell her what you'll be wearing. Or, if you don't want me to do that, because this one day is not that big a deal for you, I won't and maybe you can modify your dress."

If he says, "No, mom, I cannot change how I dress on Thanksgiving. This is who I am," you've got to honor that. Then you need to call grandma and prepare her by saying, "Mom, this is what you are going to see and I understand if it upsets you or troubles you, but James is still your grandson and I expect you to be there for him on Thanksgiving."

On the other hand, your son might not want to deal with grandma so may be willing to go along with your request to dress conventionally for a day. You can point out this isn't a permanent decision but a decision made for a specific circumstance on a specific day.

But whatever his final decision, you must go along with it.

Thanksgiving dinner is one example of a time when you may feel torn between your child and another family member. Time and again, you will need to choose between your child's comfort and that of others. The discomfort of others may have *some* consequences for your child, but your child's discomfort could have far more serious repercussions for him and for your relationship with him.

It bears repeating: Your first priority at all times should be your child's needs. If you don't put his needs first, you will have an isolated, alienated, at-risk child.

My child wants to be a different gender.

Say your son, who is a boy biologically, says, "I feel like a girl. I've always felt like a girl and I always will." Depending on your child's age, the most important thing is to keep talking to see if the feeling persists. If it continues until he's in his late teens, then he should talk to a therapist to make an informed decision about how to proceed. In the meantime, you can engage him in dialogue by asking some of the following questions:

- What makes you feel that way?
- Do you always feel that or only at certain times?
- Why do you think it would be easier to be a girl or if you had a female body?
- What is it about that body that would make it easier?

Your aim in exploring his answers to these questions is to sort out whether your child is truly transgendered. Keep the following two questions in the back of your mind during your discussions:

1. Is your child responding to a narrow definition of gender? Is your son saying, "I like to sew and only girls sew, so that's why I want to be a girl"? Is your daughter saying, "I love football and only guys can play, so I want to be a boy"?

   If this appears to be so, then at some point, ask your son point blank: "Is one of your reasons for wanting to be a girl because you love to sew?" If he says "yes," then review the suggestions at the end of Chapter 3 for how to give your son a broad positive view of masculinity. Ask your daughter a similar question related to her interests and then discuss with her an inclusive definition of femininity, also based on the suggestions at the end of Chapter 3.

2. Is he responding to sexual feelings that he doesn't know how to handle in any other way? For example, is he thinking, I'm attracted to boys, therefore I need to become a girl to actualize that attraction?

   If so, he may be LGB, he may be in denial about being LGB, or he may be questioning his orientation. The next chapter will give you information about how to handle a child who is questioning his orientation.

If neither of these questions seems to apply to your child's situation, then he may be genuinely dealing with issues around his gender identity. These issues need to be dealt with in a professional setting. If your child has consistently identified as a member of the opposite sex for at least six months, I recommend a consultation with a mental health professional who has an understanding of the transgender experience. He or she can help your child explore his issues and help you understand what he's going through.

My child wants to change his name.

Although it may be difficult for you to begin calling your daughter Susan by a boy's name, such as Frank or Tim, it is an introductory way for her to begin to try out what it feels like to be and be seen as the other gender. Anybody can change his name anytime. It's not permanent, like surgery.

This can be an important part of the transitioning process. Often people will actually realize they don't want to change their sex, but only some aspects of expected gender roles, just by going through the experiment of changing their name and seeing what that feels like. He can always change it back.

I once was involved in an organization with a twenty-two-year-old college graduate named Harry who started going by the name Sabina. (His parents don't know about the name change. They still call him Harry.) At our meetings, we put nameplates in front of everyone. He asked that his nameplate say Sabina. Of course, we honored his wishes. When he saw the nameplate in front of his seat, he started crying. He said, "It just means so much to me that you're willing to call me by what I want to be called."

It is rare for transgendered people to feel validated for who they really are. This young man was so touched to receive a nameplate that matched what he wanted to be called that he actually burst into tears at the meeting.

My child wants to begin hormones or have
reassignment surgery.

The decision to have sex reassignment surgery (what used to be called "the sex change operation") is obviously an enormous one. There are far more young people in need of help in finding a way to relate to their gender in a manner authentic to their own feelings than young people who are actually looking for reassignment surgery. Even though your child may express this desire, it's important that he and you obtain as much information about these processes as you can before making any final decisions. Never begin this process without medical and psychological counseling.

Taking hormones and undergoing surgery are serious, life-changing actions. Because the surgery is irreversible, most experts advise young people to hold off until they've gone through their biological adolescence and may be better able to make such a decision. As Verna Eggleston, the former Executive Director of the Hetrick-Martin Institute, the nation's largest social service agency serving LGBT youth, once put it, "I tell the children that they need to have one puberty at a time."

That said, however, the decision to have surgery should be made on an individual basis. Say you have a male child who is very feminine and has been expressing this clearly since age five in a real, conscious way and you are supportive of his expressing himself in this way. It's probably a good thing not to make this child go through another ten years of torture. In cases like this, androgen suppression may be advisable for some male-to-female youths to help prevent the effects of testosterone that will make the transition more difficult later on.

As a way to begin the process and to test the waters as a different gender, you might suggest a name change. You could say, "Surgery is a very big step and is probably not the right thing for you to do physically now, but there are other things you can do, like go by a name that feels more authentic to you." Let him live as the other gender for a while and then see if he still desires surgery.

Sometimes hormones are necessary to facilitate living as the other sex while learning how to express safely one's gender identity. Taking cross-sex hormones is not as dangerous as it might seem, providing it's done under medical supervision with a practitioner experienced in transgender medicine. Sometimes just hormones can alleviate the frustration and pressure of the transgender experience and even relieve the desire for surgery, though in other cases hormones may confirm the appropriateness of surgery, too.

In the meantime, spend time talking about the following areas with your child as you and he seriously think about surgery. It's a good idea to have these discussions in the presence of a mental health professional, who is not emotionally involved in your family. The following questions are a good springboard for your talk.

- how does he envision his life in five, ten, fifteen years?
- what are his dreams and goals?
- what will it means for his body to go through this kind of transition?
- what are the physical consequences?
- what are the implications for the family?

Contact the Harry Benjamin International Gender Dysphoria Association (www.HBIGDA.org)*, which established the Standards of Care required for transsexual medical treatments,

---

* Harry Benjamin was an endocrinologist who pioneered the use of hormones in sex reassignment. He popularized the term "transsexual" when he published a book in 1965 called *The Transsexual Phenomenon*. He was understanding and supportive of trans people and encouraged many other compassionate professionals to work with transpeople to ease their suffering.

for guidance in this area. These standards, which are general guidelines, include the following:

- being at least sixteen years of age
- having had the desire to change sex for a number of years
- being in the care of a therapist for at least a year.

Each case, however, must be individually evaluated.

Sometimes when teens find out they can change their sex, they'll decide immediately, "That's it, that's what I want and I know it." Nothing will sway them. They need to understand they can't just do that. Some find ways to get hormones on the street or from the Internet, and try to begin their gender reassignment on their own, with no medical or counseling advice.

If you find out your child has begun hormones on his own, you need to sit down with him and explain that this is a very serious step with very serious repercussions, and that some hormones cause permanent, irreversible changes. Find out exactly which hormone he is taking, at what dosage and for how long he has been taking it. Then consult a physician familiar with such matters.

Black market hormones may not be pharmaceutically pure, or may not contain the proper dosage. If your child is getting hormones on the street be sure he is not sharing needles. This is one of the ways HIV/AIDS and other serious diseases can be transmitted.

SHOULD MY TRANS TEEN BE IN THERAPY?

If you are thinking of sending your child into therapy so he will accept his biological sex, you are sending him for the wrong reason. Just as therapists cannot change a child's sexual orientation, they cannot make your child's biological sex and gender correspond, nor can they reverse his transgender tendencies. ·

But therapists can help your child come to terms with who he is and help him feel comfortable about that. They can also help trans teens handle the rejection and ostracism they face at school. It is very difficult to learn in a hostile environment. As we know, the social scene can be brutal for trans teens. Given the priority attached to conforming to traditional gender norms in our society, even the slightest deviation can bring swift retribution from one's peers. For those students who identify as transgender, the pain can be even greater than for LGB students. A therapist can lend extra support and provide needed coping skills.

In Chapter 10, I discuss in detail how to find a therapist and what to ask when you interview a therapist for your teen. Please review those guidelines. In addition, use the following questions as a guide to determine how comfortable and experienced the therapist is with transgendered youth. Feel free to add your own questions as well.

- What kind of professional training have you had to work with adolescents, trans people, or both?
- What is your past experience with trans people and with youth in particular?
- What is your position with respect to transgender issues? You should look for somebody who says basically that he or she is aware that people have different experiences with respect to gender and that not everybody feels the same way.

There are several ways to find a good gender therapist.

1. Ask for a referral from your physician, clergy, family counselor or another therapist who doesn't specialize in gender issues but may know someone who does.

2. Ask parents at a PFLAG meeting for referrals.

3. Contact national referral resources in the Resources section at the back of the book.

FINDING SUPPORT FOR YOUR TRANS TEEN

More than even LGB youth, many trans teens feel as if they're the "only one." They feel totally alone and isolated. They can't imagine that anyone else is going through what they're experiencing. They have no place where they belong or where they can be themselves. That's why it's so crucial for your child to connect with other trans teens.

Following are five ways for him to begin connecting with other trans teens and making personal contact with them:

1. Seek out a gay-straight alliance at his school, if it has one. Depending on the school, there may or may not be other trans teens in the gay-straight alliance but the organization will connect him with LGB teens, who should be more accepting than straight teens and who may also know other trans teens in town.

2. Ask other parents at PFLAG meetings for local resources.

3. Check out web sites, geared to trans teens listed in the Resources section. These are places where your child can express himself freely, remain anonymous and feel accepted.

4. Watch movies like *Boys Don't Cry.*

5. Read books on trans teens recommended in the Resources section of this book.

FINDING SUPPORT FOR YOURSELF

Just as your child needs to surround himself with others who are transgendered, you need to realize that you are not the only parent going through this. I can't stress enough the importance of going to PFLAG meetings. You will find other parents who have faced the same issues personally, who have found ways to cope with a trans child and who have helped him face challenges at school and with his peers.

It is also important to stay connected to friends and family members who are supportive. You know who they are. This is not the time to be with people who are judgmental of you or your child—even if they are a close relative. If you hear critical comments, you may have to be blunt and say something like, "This is not good for me to hear now. I need to get off the phone." Or you may have to refuse to see someone for a while if you feel the relationship is undermining your personal process of accepting your transgendered child. That may mean saying, "I need some time to myself right now. I think it's best if I don't see you for a while. I have things I need to work out and I need to do it by myself." Then find other PFLAG parents and discuss with them how they handled friends and family members who weren't supportive.

While you are finding support for yourself, do some reading by other parents of trans teens. You'll find a list of books in the Resources section at the back of the book. Reading these books will show you that it is possible to live a full and happy life after changing one's sex or being transgendered in any of the myriad ways trans people experience their lives.

DEFINITIONS

Cross-dresser: One who dresses, either in public or private, in clothing that society assigns to the opposite sex. Cross-dressing is not an indication of one's sexual orientation or gender identity. The formerly used term "transvestite" is now considered offensive by some, because it implies a particular type of distressed behavior that is not common to all who cross-dress.

Female to Male (FTM): A person who was born with a female body, but identifies as or feels male, and who takes on or accepts the sex, gender, or both of a male either through hormones, surgery, mannerisms, dress, behavior, etc.

Gender: The socially and culturally defined behaviors assigned to females and males based on their biological sex. That defines masculine and feminine.

Gender Reassignment Surgery: A surgical procedure that modifies one's primary and/or secondary sex characteristics through surgery. This process was formerly called a "sex change operation," a phrase now considered offensive, because the surgery does not change their sex but reassigns them to the gender they feel they belong in.

Intersexed: At least one in 2,000 children are born with some degree of ambiguity or reversal regarding their primary and/or secondary sex characteristics. In these cases, medical personnel cannot easily label the child "boy" or "girl." Some of these children receive cosmetic surgery so that the child's genitalia conform to societal and familial expectations of "normalcy," even though such surgeries are not medically necessary and can damage the child's reproductive organs. The number of children born with some degree of intersexuality is difficult to estimate. Though intersexed people are opposed to the word "hermaphrodite" because it is misleading and stigmatizing, it continues to be widely used.

Male to Female (MTF): A person who was born with a male body, but identifies as or feels female, and who takes on or accepts the sex, gender, or both of a female either through hormones, surgery, mannerisms, dress, behavior, etc.

Sex: How society classifies us, based on our reproductive biology. When we talk about sex, we use the words female and male.

Transgender: An umbrella term for all those who may choose not to or are otherwise unable to conform to society's often stereotypical notions of gender expression, including transsexuals, cross-dressers, Two Spirit people, and drag queens and kings. This term refers to a wide range of people who either do not identify with or cannot conform to the gender roles assigned to them based on their biological sex.

Transsexual: Individuals who do not identify with their birth-assigned sex, and sometimes alter their bodies to reconcile their gender identity and their physical body and/or biological sex.

Chapter Seven

THE QUESTIONING
TEEN

WHILE YOU MAY SEE your teen struggling with issues related to school and friends, you may not see evidence of her difficulties with her sexual identity. Yet this is much more difficult than anything else she is coping with.

And she may be facing it alone.

The fact is, when it comes to sexual orientation, many more teens grapple with the issue than "just" those who are LGBT.

I knew from a very early age that I was attracted to boys, but in the world in which I was raised, this simply was not possible. I was a good boy and homosexuality was definitely bad, so there was no way I could hold onto my image of myself as a good boy if I were also a homosexual. All I knew about homosexuals was that they lived in San Francisco and were doing bad things. They were certainly not in North Carolina, where I was growing up.

I was confused, because I knew what I was feeling, but I also knew that it "wasn't possible." That made sense to my thirteen-year-old mind. I had heard various myths through the grapevine: that you might be attracted to boys but those feelings will go away or you'll meet the right girl someday and you'll be fine. I hoped and prayed that that would happen to me.

Many teenagers find it impossible to mesh their own internal feelings, which they sense are true and right, with all of society's negative images of homosexuality that run through their heads, as I did. They are so scared and unsure that they allow their fears to overwhelm what they know to be true about themselves. Other teens struggle with their orientation differently. For example, some girls think they're in love with their best friend and just want to snuggle with her, while others are fascinated by their girlfriend in almost an obsessive way. Their adoration may cause them to question their orientation.

No matter what their particular struggle, however, their behavior, orientation and identity are not in sync. At least one part does not mesh with the others, so they try on different kinds of behaviors to help them figure out what feels right to them. They desperately want to feel whole, but they don't know where to turn.

They feel as though they're stranded in the middle of the ocean in a rowboat without a rudder—all alone. They can't identify with an LGBT community or a straight community. There is no place where they feel they belong and can simply be themselves.

Questioning teens are at high risk for problems. Because they are isolated, they can easily become depressed and turn to drugs and alcohol to numb the pain, or develop an eating disorder as a way to gain some control over their lives. The longer there is a disconnect between who they really are and what they're doing, the more serious the situation becomes.

Reducing their sense of isolation is the goal, and this is best done through the kind of nonjudgmental and open communication we talked about in Chapter 1. To be able to do that, though, you need to understand the nature of their struggle. In this chapter, we'll explore the three types of questioning that occur so you can recognize your child's particular challenge. I'll alert you to the signs that your child may be questioning her orientation, and tell you what you can do if you suspect she is questioning. I'll also talk about experimentation, a common occurrence among questioning teens.

As you read this chapter, keep in mind that all of these youth are in a transition stage. Some will turn out gay or lesbian, some will recognize they are straight; some will be transgendered and some bisexual. The reality is, all of these teens are genuinely questioning their orientation or gender identity. But they are doing it totally alone. They desperately need support—your support, the support of other family members and friends who care about them, and the support of their school and community.

The kind of support that questioning teens want is space in which they are not asked to immediately put a label on themselves, where they can talk about feelings on Monday and then say the exact opposite on Tuesday and yet not feel judged or that they are being inconsistent. If they do contradict what they said the next day, they want someone to say to them, "You're not crazy. That's okay."

This situation can be confusing for a parent. To help you understand what's going on—without judging your child—simply note the behavior. You can say, "Gosh, this is different from what you said before and I'm really curious to understand why. It's okay with me if you have changed your mind or your point of view, but I'm just trying to make sure I understand what you're thinking. Can you fill me in here?"

Young people don't want to be pushed into a corner or made to feel they have to decide or justify their feelings or their inconsistencies. Questioning teens need permission to *not* come up with an answer until they are ready, which is hard for parents, who want to know their teen's orientation so that they can do the right thing.

A SPECTRUM OF BEHAVIORS

It may surprise you to learn that young people come to know their sexual orientation at a very young age; one study found that most recognize their orientation around the age of eleven and a half. As we discussed in Chapter 2, orientation, which is the attraction one feels toward either or both sexes, is not something that others can cause you to change. But there is a broad spectrum of sexual behaviors—the sex acts one engages in—that people can experience over the course of their lifetime. Sexual identity—how others see you and how you see yourself—can also change. People may come to terms with their orientation and make decisions around behavior and identity at many different points, as we discussed earlier.

Questioning youth are easier to understand if you think about the continuum of sexual behaviors ranging from heterosexual to bisexual to homosexual that we discussed earlier. Many straight teens have same-sex experiences and many LGBT teens have opposite-sex experiences. Back in the '40s and '50s, Kinsey found that 37 percent of men and 10 percent of women had had same-sex experiences as teens, so there's nothing new about this. Those figures may be higher today, because we have more sexual freedom and more acceptance of a variety of lifestyles.

EXPERIMENTATION

The teen years are a time for adolescents to figure out who they are, what they like and what turns them on. They try different styles of clothes, cut or dye their hair in unconventional ways, and listen to all kinds of music. It's natural for all teens—whether LGBT, straight or questioning—to experiment sexually either with the opposite sex or the same sex.

Yet experimentation may still trouble you, as it does many

parents. Your disapproval will not stop your child's behavior, however. (It probably didn't stop you, did it?) But if your child feels your displeasure, it will only compound the dissatisfaction she may already feel about herself. As you know, when children's self-esteem declines, they are more at risk for problems. They may fall into a depression, cut themselves, overeat or undereat, or lose interest in school and their courses.

You may be wondering why teens need to experiment. I've found there are four reasons that this happens:

1. Some experiment because they're bisexual.
2. Some do it because they're homosexual and want desperately to be heterosexual and are "trying to get it right."
3. Some experiment with the same sex because they become overwhelmed by feelings of emotional closeness and then physical intimacy just happens, even when it's not their true orientation.
4. Some teens do it because it's interesting and fun.

Jane, a high school student, was shocked by what she observed one night after a party, as you may be. She had just told her best friend that she thought she might be a lesbian. Jane recalls, "Three girls—all straight—came home with me and we drank a little bit. We were sitting on my roof and two of them were like 'Hey, want to see what we can do?' And they kissed and then we all kissed different people.

"It was astonishing to me," she continues, "because supposedly all of those girls just happen to kiss each other all the time. It was just something they did. They would just get drunk and kiss each other. I just had no idea that this was happening. My friend and I exchanged looks like, 'Oh, my God, if they only knew that you actually liked girls,' but that was kind of interesting to me. I don't think any of those people would have considered themselves bisexual or queer or whatever."

Jane is probably right—for now. If your child is experimenting with the same sex, you may wonder if that's an indication that
she's LGBT.

The reality is, if teens do experiment with the same sex there
is a possibility that they'll identify as LGBT. But many, many
more people experiment than end up as LGBT. There is a corre-
lation, but not a causal effect.

DISCUSSING EXPERIMENTATION

When kids start to experiment sexually or become sexually active, we often think of them as grown-up or mature. But remember: they are still young—no matter how big they are or how
sophisticated they look. More than at any other point, they need
you, because when they get involved sexually for the first time,
they are vulnerable in a way that they haven't felt before.

If your teen wants to experiment, probably nothing is going to
stop her no matter what you say. In many cases, you may never
know. But you must assume experimentation is a possibility and
proceed accordingly. Just as you talk with your child about the
dangers of drugs, whether or not your child is using them, I recommend that you sit down and talk with her about sexual experimentation. Experimentation can be just as harmful as doing
drugs if a child is vulnerable.

In your discussion, try to set aside your own moral judgments and make sure your teen has accurate information about
safe sex.

Here are five important points to make:

1. Acknowledge up front that this discussion is awkward
   and uncomfortable for you and probably for your teen,
   and that's okay. You can say, "This is difficult for me to
   talk about. It's probably difficult for you to hear from me

as well, but I read the statistics and I know what goes on. I don't want you to think I'm trying to figure out what you're doing or that I'm judging what you're doing. That is not my goal here." In this way, you're upfront about your own discomfort, you explain why you're having the conversation and you make it clear that your purpose is educational, not judgmental.

2. Then, talk about your concerns. Preface the discussion by saying, "Look, I'm not saying you do or you don't, but I know that a lot of young people experiment sexually. Whether or not you do is probably outside my control, but there are some things you need to know if you're experimenting, or do so in the future. Ignoring them can cost you your life, or cause things to happen that you may not be ready for, like being a parent." Then, talk about the dangers of unprotected sex and how to protect herself. See the Resources section for recommended books on this topic.

3. Address experimentation as a health issue, not a moral one. Get the message across that regardless of whom she's with, she needs to understand what's safe and what's not. If you find out that your child is engaging in same-sex experimentation, you don't want to say, "Oh, my God, don't you know you're going to catch AIDS?" That sounds like a moral judgment. A teen will hear, my parent doesn't approve of me, my parent thinks what I'm doing is wrong. Then she will withdraw from the whole conversation. Instead, say, "Honey, I love you. But some sexual behaviors can be dangerous, and you need to protect yourself—no matter whom you're with."

4. Acknowledge that this information may not be needed now but she may need it in the future. You can say, "This information may not be relevant to what is happening

with you right now. It may not be relevant for five or ten years, but I would rather you have it sooner rather than later."

5. Stress often the crucial reason that you are having this discussion. Say something like, "I want you to know that my bottom line is: regardless of how I feel about what you're doing, I am discussing this with you because I love you and I want you to be healthy. I want you to understand that it is never, ever okay to engage in unsafe sexual behavior. Not because it is morally wrong or right, but because I want to see you grow up to be a happy, healthy adult. As we discussed, serious consequences can result from engaging in unsafe behavior that can stop that from happening."

TYPES OF QUESTIONING

I've divided youth who are questioning their orientation into three categories for the purpose of explaining them. In reality, there are no such distinct divisions. The categories overlap. Your child may be in more than one category at the same time, may shift among them at any point, or show bits and pieces of each type. Each has elements that are both conscious and unconscious, which means that your child may not be in touch with what she's doing or why she's doing it.

I've identified each type with a capsule quotation that sums up the turmoil, followed by a personal story. You'll probably recognize your child in one of these stories. The section that follows will give you suggestions for how to cope with a questioning teen. The three types are:

1. "I can't be. You mean I'm bad?" These teens are confused because deep down on an unconscious level, they

know who they are, but it terrifies them and they don't know how to proceed with it.

When they suspect they might be LGBT, they take on the burden of society's homophobia and denigrate themselves. But these negative images do not fit the image they have of themselves. This discrepancy throws them into a state of chaos. They also feel totally alone and misunderstood, certain that no one else could possibly feel the way they do.

Jared realized he was attracted to boys in his sophomore year of high school. But he also knew he couldn't possibly be gay. He said, "I didn't know what that was, because to me, gay was something I wasn't. I knew I liked boys but for me, being gay would be something weird and I was ordinary. So I guess I was questioning the fact that word applied to me, because I was just myself."

Stereotypes definitely played a role in his negative view of homosexuals. "I thought they were just going to be everything—from glamourous to child molesters— I'm sad to say, but that's how I kind of thought about them. That is what society tells you."

Jared was totally confused: he would develop a crush on a guy and get excited, and then all the negative things about gay men would come tumbling to his mind: That can't be me. I can't really feel that way. There was no one he could talk to. He was sure no one else felt as he did.

He felt so depressed and alienated that for several months he wanted to die. Finally, he opened up to Mr. Bridges, the school guidance counselor. "I just bawled my eyes out with him, and told him I didn't want to live any more," he remembers. Mr. Bridges introduced Jared to a student who was a lesbian. "When I met her, it was just like a whole new world opened up. It was like, Oh, my God, there's someone else. I remember just feeling so alone before that and after I met her, my world changed." Very slowly after that, he started telling other people he was gay. His depression lifted.

Jared's depression resulted in part from internalized homophobia, a situation that many LGBTQ youth experience when they internalize society's stigmas and stereotypes about homosexuality. Growing up feeling different and being criticized for that difference, they personalize the criticism, as well as society's negative views of LGBT people. They end up feeling ashamed and dejected, having absorbed society's rejection of them by rejecting themselves. Once Jared had someone positive to identify with who was LGBT, he began to feel better about himself.

2. "I love my best friend. Does that mean I'm gay?" These are the teens who are engaging in behaviors that don't mesh with their orientation or with what society tells them they should be.

As teens sort through social pressures and their personal feelings, they may fall all along the spectrum of sexual behaviors. Don't automatically give your child a label because of what you see. If your son is having homosexual experiences, it doesn't necessarily mean he's gay. He may or may not be. Or, if you suspect your daughter is a lesbian and she comes home with a boyfriend, don't necessarily assume she's straight.

Many teenagers become infatuated with their best (same-sex) friend. This happens particularly when they confuse homosexual and homosocial behavior. In high school, girls tend to hang out with other girls and boys, with other boys. That's called "homosocial" behavior: socializing with people of the same gender. Sometimes girls and boys, however, become confused because they know what their homosocial feelings are—this is my best friend, I love her/him to death, and she/he is more important to me than anyone else—but they don't know what that means. Does that mean I'm LGBT? Does that mean other people will call me an LGBT?

Stephan was a dancer who was emotionally attached to his best friend, Will. One Saturday night, he slept over at Will's house and they had sex. Stephan was blown away, "Oh, my God," he thought. "I must be gay. What do I do now?" Will reinforced his feeling by telling him, "If you feel this way about me and you wanted to have sex with me, you must be gay." Stephan also got the message from the larger culture that boys who are interested in dance are gay. He drew the conclusion, "I must be gay, after all, because certainly everybody in the world seems to expect me to be gay and I'm emotionally attached to my best friend. I just had sex with him." But this didn't jibe with what Stephan felt deep down, which was that he was ordinarily attracted to girls.

Anyone can do something—sexual or not—that's outside of the realm of what they usually do. You may run a four-minute mile one time and never do it again. It just happens. Sometimes, because of the heat of the moment or the emotional connection involved, people can do something that is not what they'd typically do. That was the case here. Today, Stephan is married with a family.

This kind of homosocial behavior means something different to men and women. Women often conflate sexual attraction with emotional attachment. Even for men, sexuality can be an expression of closeness or just fun. So, it's not such a surprise to me that teens act out their affection for their friend with actual sexual behavior. As a parent, you may be baffled by the behavior but you may need to sit tight and let the situation evolve.

3. "I think I'm gay. I think I'm not. I think I'm gay . . ."
   These teens are questioning their orientation for all or
   some of the above reasons. They just can't figure out
   where they fit on the spectrum and are having trouble
   sorting out their feelings in light of the negative messages they receive from the world around them. Their
   questioning is born of the fear that comes from homophobia.

   Like Joni, they're completely perplexed about their
sexual orientation and don't know if they're straight, bi
or gay. A college student today, Joni found herself becoming obsessed with different girls—not particularly
in a sexual way, but just fascinated by them when she
was in high school. She'd get nervous when she saw
them or she'd purposely have a cigarette in certain
places to bump into them. Female teachers had always
intrigued her. Although she never dated guys, she
hooked up with them and had crushes on boys in middle
school.

   At the end of her junior year of high school, Joni came
out to her parents after she attended a gay-straight alliance meeting at her school. But once she had said the
word lesbian aloud, her doubts began to set in. She told
her parents it wasn't true. Her dad tried to be understanding, but her mother was frantic and confused. A
few days later, she found that Joni had visited gay web
sites and confronted her. Joni recalls, "She pulled me
into her room and she was like, 'You need to tell me—are
you gay?' Of course I had no idea if I was gay or not. I was
kind of confused about it. So I said, 'Yes, no, maybe, I
don't know. Why are you asking me this?' It was really
awful."

   After that brief discussion, they had a kind of truce
where they didn't discuss her orientation. Yet Joni

needed someone to talk to. Six months later she came out to her mother as a bisexual. Her mother told her that bisexuality didn't exist, that she was either gay or straight. Joni says, "She honestly—deep in her heart— believes that I am straight and that this is just a phase, which is definitely possible. I know that I am attracted to girls, but it's possible that I will end up marrying a man. I definitely don't rule that out, but I needed her to respect my decision and my identity in high school."

Her dad took a low-key approach and told her it didn't matter what she was, that he was proud of her, and yet he pressed her for answers, too. At one point he asked her, "How are you doing with this whole gay thing?" She recalls, "It made me so nervous to talk about it with them because I wasn't sure, and I didn't know, and I was so back and forth. Am I gay, am I straight? Also, if I entered a gay culture there are a bunch of other things that would get thrown in my face: Are you butch, are you fem, are you dating, are you having sex? All this stuff. It was just a lot for me."

Joni remained conflicted throughout high school. Although today she calls herself a lesbian, she remains ambivalent about the label. She and her parents still cannot discuss her orientation easily. "A part of me thinks maybe they're right. Maybe I really am straight. All my friends are straight except for my girlfriend and most people don't know we're dating. I have a really hard time with people who identify themselves only as gay. I identify myself like me, Joni, not like Joni-gay.

"I've definitely picked up on my parents' homophobia and I have a little bit of internalized homophobia, which is too bad. I don't hate gay people. Obviously, I don't hate myself for being gay, but I don't want to identify as a gay person either."

Clearly, Joni is still struggling to figure out "this whole gay thing." Her parents constantly questioning her—and interrogating her—about her orientation created doubts in Joni's mind. Their rejection of any orientation other than heterosexuality and their insistence on answers NOW undermined her confidence, rather than supported her.

COPING WITH A QUESTIONING TEEN

If a child is shamed or silenced, in ways subtle or overt, because of the stigma attached to a label, that can drive her away or lead her to withdraw, become depressed or strike out in anger.

Here are guidelines for coping with a teen who is questioning her orientation in any of the above ways:

• Acknowledge with her that at some point in their lives many people engage in behaviors or have identities that conflict with their orientation. Tell her that it's not unusual for people who are basically heterosexual to have a homosexual experience, or for people who are LGBT to be identified by others as being straight. It's typical and normal.

• Tell her that once she figures out what her orientation is, she should try to engage in behaviors that will develop an identity that is consistent with that. Suggest that she reflect on the following two questions:

1. Am I really being myself, or am I being what other people want me to be?

2. Why do I act the way I do? Is it because it's the way that I want to act, or because I think my Mom wants me to act this way, or because the kids in my

school want me to act a certain way, or because I've
been taught to act this way?

• Remind her that it never works to try and act like someone
you are not. Say to your child again and again, "Be honest about
who you are" or "Be true to yourself"—and mean it. Children
know their parents and can sense when they are saying something heartfelt and when they are just saying the appropriate
words.

• Draw on your child's own experiences. Was there a time
when she was younger that she tried acting in a certain way to
win friends or be more popular? What was the result of that? You
could say, "Remember back in third grade when you thought
having a Polo shirt would make everybody like you and you saved
all your allowance money and bought one and people felt the
same way about you the next day? This is like that."

• Don't press your teen for an answer or constantly question
whether she's LGBT. She sincerely doesn't know. Pushing her to
identify as LGBT or straight only puts more pressure on her and
will alienate her from you, because she knows that you're not accepting her answer and she wants to give you a satisfactory reply.

• Don't criticize her. She has probably taken on some of
society's homophobia and feels negative about herself already.
She doesn't need more condemnation.

• Accept whatever label she uses. It's how she feels at the
present moment. Try not to project into the future. The label
may change, or it may not. She deserves your respect today.

• As always, try to develop the qualities that create an open
atmosphere in your home.

• Let her know that you love her and accept her for who she
is, whether she's LGBT or straight. A lot of parents assume that
their children know they're loved. But, being raised in a homophobic society, young people who are questioning their orientation tend to assume the worst. They don't assume that you still

think they're great. They don't know that you still value them for being a good soccer player or a good flutist. They may think that their questioning and struggles just wiped all of that away.

Just as the advertising people do, take a very simple message and repeat it over and over again. Say it out loud, even if you feel like a broken record. Tell her, "I love you" again and again. Some days say, "I love you just the way you are." Also remind her, "I trust that you'll work this out. Wherever you end up is okay by me."

SIGNS OF QUESTIONING

It may be difficult for you to know whether your child is questioning her orientation, because these youths tend to be heavily guarded and do not talk openly about their struggles with their parents. But there are signs that can alert you that your child may be questioning her sexual orientation.

Keep in mind, though, that these signs—a sudden change in weight, appearance or risky behavior—are the result of a complex interplay of factors. You cannot automatically assume that these behaviors mean that your child is questioning her orientation.

I wish I could give you a unique marker or magic bullet that would immediately tell you that your child is questioning her orientation, but no such thing exists.

A sudden change in behavior can also be a sign of adolescent depression and an indication of sexual abuse. You must evaluate each sign in light of what you know about your child and what else is going on in the family and in your child's life.

The four signs of questioning include:

1. A sudden change in behavior, particularly risky behavior. This may include staying out late, starting to smoke, or reading hard-core porn magazines. New risky behavior

may be due to the influence of a new group of friends, or it could mean that your child feels so alone and dejected that she doesn't care what happens to her.

One young man, who suspected he had sexual feelings towards people of the same gender, spent several years trying to change those feelings and desires. He never thought he was gay, but only that something was wrong with him for not being straight. At age sixteen without the support of family, friends or teachers, he turned to pot and alcohol to escape his feelings of depression.

He recalls, "What started as a simple curiosity of what alcohol and cigarettes tasted and felt like, soon became a realization that such products could be used to make me happy, to escape the depression that was plaguing my life. I soon surrounded myself with a new group of friends, who supported my habits and by the beginning of my senior year in high school, I was having a shot of alcohol before school, and skipping out midday to drink by the river. I started smoking pot, originally for the sole purpose of helping me sleep at night, to avoid the hours of crying myself to sleep and contemplating suicide. Before long, I turned to stronger drugs—acid, speed, ecstasy, cocaine."

2. A sudden change in appearance, including a dramatic change in style of dress or a sudden weight gain or loss. Teens struggling with their orientation often gain weight, building a fortress around them to obscure their biological characteristics and ward off advances by anyone—male or female.

Joan, fifteen, a family friend, gained fifty pounds throughout the tenth grade. While she had dated boys pretty steadily up until that time, she stopped dating and also cut herself off from other activities, including her all-time favorite, dance. Joan also began skipping school and her teachers expressed concern over her erratic behavior and her plummeting grades. At a family get-together, Joan took me aside and confided that she thought she might be bisexual.

Around the same time, Joan's mother also approached me, expressing concern over Joan's behavior. She suspected that something was up in the area of sexual identity, but did not know how to bring it up with Joan. I advised Joan's mother not to press her about her sexual identity, but just to be supportive and let her know that she is willing to discuss anything that Joan might have on her mind. In the meantime, I urged Joan's mother to read and educate herself, go to PFLAG meetings and talk to friends, so that she could be more open-minded and in a positive place when the time came to talk.

3. A change in communication with peers. When a teen who is usually sociable withdraws from her friends or stops going out on weekends, that may indicate that she no longer feels comfortable with her old friends—possibly because they're straight and she's questioning her orientation. On the other hand, when a teen who normally stays home and studies suddenly starts going out every night, that may be a sign that she has found a group of friends, at last, with whom she feels compatible.

Maria and a large gang of girlfriends were inseparable all through middle school and into high school. Her sophomore year, she dropped everybody but Katie. The two of them would come home after school and hang out in Maria's room with the door closed for hours. The other girls stopped calling. Maria's mother grew concerned about what this behavior meant.

If you notice similar changes in behavior, handle this by talking about what you've observed. You can say, "I notice you're spending a lot of time with Katie" or "I notice the phone hasn't rung in weeks. Has something happened?" Then let your child respond. You don't want to say, "What do you mean—spending all your time alone with Katie in your room?" That will put your child on the defensive and make her clam up.

4. Any obsessive behavior, such as more frequent, secretive use of the Internet, excessive television watching and obsessive dating. Such behaviors can be a cover for anxiety and a way for young people to bury themselves in mindless activity and suppress uncomfortable impulses and feelings.

When youths spend a lot of time on the Internet, it may mean they are finding it hard to identify people in their daily lives with whom they feel comfortable and are turning to the online world to find companionship. This isn't a bad thing, as having someone to talk to— even via a keyboard—is better than feeling completely alone and isolated.

This is a generation that just plain feels more at home socializing online than we do, and thus doing so is hardly abnormal behavior. But when coupled with a sudden change in social behavior (dropping all their friends at school, for example), it may mean that they are using the Internet to deal with social difficulties, which can include those brought on by questioning their sexual orientation.

If you notice your son logging a lot of hours online, simply note the behavior: "I see you're spending a a lot of time online lately." Let your son take it from there.

The one thing all these scenarios have in common is that each provides a way for the child to isolate herself. Youth can be both alienated by others and they also have a huge hand in alienating themselves. That is why it is so important for parents to be attuned to a child's changing habits and interests.

CHECKING OUT YOUR SUSPICIONS

When you notice any of these changes in your child's behavior, note the behavior as I illustrated above, and then open the door a bit more by sending her a signal that you are receptive to talking. You can say, "Maybe I'm overreacting, but these are some of the reasons that have occurred to me about why people sometimes change in this way." Then give her a list of possible reasons.

For example, if you notice that your teen suddenly doesn't want to go to school anymore, you could say something like, "Sometimes people don't want to go to school anymore because they're bored or they're not interested in what they are studying. Sometimes they feel out of place and they don't have any friends. Sometimes they have discovered things about themselves that make them feel like they don't belong anymore—like their family doesn't have as much money as other families, or they may be confused by sexual feelings they hadn't expected to have—so they don't feel like they fit in with everyone else," and then list two or three more reasons.

Then, say to your child, "I'm wondering if any of these seem to make sense to you and you want to talk about them, or if there's something else I haven't thought of?"

Here are the four steps for checking out your suspicions:

1. Estimate the top three or four reasons that may be causing the behavior. Make sure you put questioning sexual orientation in the middle, not at the beginning or the end, and also leave the door open that there may be other things you haven't thought of. That signals to your

child a little more directly that you know that sexual orientation could be a reason and that you are comfortable talking about it. If you don't link the behavior explicitly to something that it is plausibly connected to, it leads young people to think that you are completely clueless and you couldn't even bring up the real reason for the behavior.

2. If your child admits that she's questioning her orientation and you are comfortable discussing it with her, then you can say, "Let's talk about your concerns."

3. If she admits she's questioning, but is not comfortable talking to you, then help her find social settings where she can be herself, such as a gay-straight alliance at school, a local youth group, web sites like Planetout.com or books and videos—if she's willing to allow you to be involved in this way. If she feels such suggestions are intrusive, then back off and let her find outlets for herself.

4. If you're not comfortable discussing her questioning, go back to Chapter 1 and review the questions for self-reflection, so you can prepare yourself for these discussions.

Some parents feel they are being intrusive by raising these questions. You are not: You are showing your child that you're open to dialogue. You have raised the issues and opened the door as much as you can without making your child feel as if her protective shell is being taken off.

Even if your child does not want to participate in the dialogue, at least she knows there is someone—a parent—who loves her enough to engage. That engagement will prevent your child from feeling alienated.

SUGGESTIONS FOR PARENTS

It is important for all teenagers to feel as if they belong, to have a peer group at school that accepts them for who they are. But questioning pre-teens and teens don't have such a place among their friends, because, of course, the issues of sexuality are fraught with anxiety at that age. Questioning teens are often totally alone and isolated. That's why your home must be a haven for them and why they need every bit of support and acceptance you can muster.

Here are five pointers for supporting your child while she sorts things out.

1. Forget labels. There is no need to put your child neatly into a box. Give her the opportunity to freely explore her orientation without insisting she find a label for herself or worrying which camp she will eventually settle in.
2. Let it be. Don't put additional pressure on your child to come to a decision about her orientation. She does not have to decide by the end of eighth grade whether she is straight or LGBT. Nor, if she hasn't had a boyfriend by eleventh grade does it mean that she's a lesbian.

    Sexuality does not come with an expiration date. Imposing artificial pressures can heighten the pressure on a young person to be inauthentic and to rush the process.

    Let your child determine the time frame. Neither you, her peers nor society needs to rush her. She will decide at a point what is right for her. Any time frame that is thrust upon her from the outside is wrong, and can lead to her engaging in behaviors that are damaging. That's the whole reason kids engage in some of the promiscuous sexual behavior: they try to experiment—

and may do it prematurely—to prove early on "I'm not gay."

And, if they get messages from parents, peers or society to make a decision by x date, they will engage in sex acts that they are not ready for intellectually or emotionally. No teen—whether straight or LGBT—should feel pressured into sex. You wouldn't want another teen to force your child, so be aware not to place the same pressure on your child.

You will eventually know, but it might not be for a while. Questioning youth need acceptance and love, not interrogation.

3. Keep in mind that what you see might not be what will be. If you think there's a lot of heterosexual sex going on, it doesn't necessarily mean your teen is straight. Likewise, if your son has a crush on his male best friend, it doesn't automatically mean he's gay. For some, their behavior is an indication of orientation, but for others, it may be experimentation or a strong emotional connection. Your job is to keep the lines of communication open so that wherever your child ends up on the spectrum of sexual identities, she will know she has a family who loves and supports her.

4. If you find it hard to talk to your child face-to-face, consider the following options as ways to lower the intensity level at home:

• Set aside a designated time to talk so that heated discussions are not going on all the time and infiltrate all your waking hours.

• Invite a third party that you both trust to be a "referee." That might create a safer place where both of you can talk through your feelings. Set up rules, such as each side getting the floor uninterrupted for three minutes at a stretch.

• Begin an email correspondence with your child. For teens who are heavily guarded, email is a less threatening way to communicate. They don't have to face you personally, and can take as much time as they need to figure out what they want to say.

If you don't already email your child, begin by sending short messages or jokes, just to get her used to getting email from you. Once you've established some back and forth, then you can get into meatier issues. You can begin a more serious email in the same way that you'd begin a discussion. Write, "I was thinking about something that happened last night," or "I'm curious about something." Then simply state your question or make a comment and say, "What do you think?" See where she takes it.

5. Lastly, remember that you have the skills you need to handle delicate situations. You have been a parent for many years. The experience you bring to being a good parent can be used to help your questioning child. There is not some separate set of skills that applies here. You know what to do. Follow your instincts.

Chapter Eight

LGBTQ YOUTH OF COLOR

"I THINK IT'S FAIR to say I grew up without any real role models," recalls Jason, an eighteen-year-old gay man. "There aren't Asian Pacific Americans on TV—Connie Chung and a few Fu Manchu rip-offs don't really count. There are even fewer gays and lesbians. Experiencing life as a double minority has given me insight into how people focus on the parts of a person rather than on the whole.

"About a year and a half ago, I came out. Being involved in a support group helped me overcome my confusion and helped me to become proud of my sexuality. But I began to distance myself from my cultural heritage. The Chinese family sees homosexuality as abnormal and immoral. This caused me to hate myself for being yellow. Reconciling and integrating my sexual identity and cultural background is a major obstacle for me."

Jason has not come out to his parents, who put a high value on Chinese traditions. He says, "This puts an incredible barrier between us. I am afraid they will be deeply hurt and confused when I decide to share this part of my life with them."

No parent wants her child to hate himself for who he is. Yet many young LGBTQ people of color, like Jason, often feel torn between what they have been taught about their culture's "traditions" and their sexual orientation. They just don't see how they can be both LGBTQ and a person of color, and be happy and accepted by the people whose affection they need and want most: their parents.

In this chapter I will use the term "of color" to refer to all people of color, which includes Arab Americans, African Americans, Asian Pacific Americans, Latino/a Americans, Native Americans, Pacific Islanders, and people of mixed race. The chapter will focus, however, on the three largest populations of people of color in the United States: African Americans, Asian Pacific Americans and Latino/a Americans.

LGBTQ teens of color face unique challenges in addition to all those faced by teens, people of color, and LGBTQ people everywhere. Not only must LGBTQ teens of color confront pervasive anti-gay bias in the broader culture, but they also face an LGBTQ culture dominated by Whites who can be ignorant or even hostile toward people of color. Add to this the fact that communities of color have many traditions that impact LGBTQ issues in different ways, and you can see how a young LGBTQ person of color faces multiple "identity" issues that teens from the dominant culture do not.

In this chapter, I'll discuss how issues specific to communities of color affect LGBTQ youth. An underlying theme of this chapter will be my encouraging you to understand that your own cultural "traditions" are not written in stone but have evolved themselves, and that this is yet another phase in that process for you, your family, and your community.

I'll give you guidelines for staying true to what is meaningful to you, while at the same time affirming your child for who he is. This is a very challenging task. We do not want LGBTQ youth to feel they have to reject either their cultural community or their LGBTQ identity, because they cannot reconcile the different parts into a unified whole.

You play a critical role in this. The most important thing a parent of an LGBTQ child of color can do is to help him find a way to develop a positive identity that embraces both his sexual orientation and his cultural heritage and integrates them in a healthy way. In this chapter, I'll discuss how you can help your child do that. I'll end the chapter with the moving story of a parent who, over time, came to accept her child's sexual orientation. Perhaps she can serve as an inspiration to you.

YOUR CULTURAL TRADITIONS

While it is simplistic and even dangerous to make generalizations about any group, I am, nonetheless, going to explore some of the specific issues LGBTQ youth from various cultures face. If you are a person of color, you, of course, know the mores and values of your own culture better than I do as a White person. But I have worked with a large number of LGBTQ teens of color over the years and those experiences have given me some insight.

Now, I'd like you to revisit your own culture with new eyes—as the parent of a LGBTQ teenager.

Keep in mind that there are great variations within each culture. The term "Asian Pacifi American" for example covers many groups that hardly see eye-to-eye on anything: Imagine a dialogue between a Muslim from the South Asian subcontinent, a Catholic from the Philippines, and a Buddhist from China about what is "Asian," and you get the idea. There are many traditions and cultures within each of the communities we'll discuss. Every culture is complex and has many facets to it. I cannot cover all the nuances, so I'm going to review some of the highlights as they pertain to your child's sexual orientation.

I am not telling you this is the way to view your culture and how it affects LGBTQ youth. Rather, I'm saying this is one way to think about how aspects of any culture might affect LGBTQ youth.

In the section that follows, I will list some values common to many of these communities and then discuss how they relate to LGBTQ issues. Of course, these values are not shared equally by all who identify with a particular culture and are sometimes shared by people who are not of color. But as you read the section that follows, try to think about how these issues might impact an LGBTQ child who does not follow the "traditional" roles and rules of your ethnic community.

African American Cultures

Among many African Americans, the following three values are often strong:

1. The prominent role of the Christian church as a bastion of the community.

2. The importance of perpetuating and raising the status of the race in the face of a hostile racist society

3. The importance of community membership as a source of support in the face of hostility

For a lot of African Americans, being LGBTQ—by which I mean the current American "gay lifestyle" of coming out and living outside heterosexual marriage with partner(s) of the same-sex—is perceived as a "White thing." That doesn't mean there haven't been LGBTQ people in African American communities. As one gay young man said, "There was always the church organist and we knew he was gay, but no one ever talked about it. There was the florist and we knew he was gay, but no one ever said a word."

What was hard for his family was how he lived differently from the stereotype of the gay organist and the gay florist: "My coming out and living with another man and talking about it was just unprecedented in my family. They weren't troubled so much

by the fact that I was gay, because they knew there were gay people. They were troubled by the way I was flaunting it. They were
like, 'Why can't you kind of just be nice and quiet like the church
organist? Why do you have to bring shame on our community?' "

This sentiment is so pervasive in African American communities that a new term has emerged: MSM—men having sex
with men. Many Black gay men will not identify as gay because
they see that as being in conflict with being Black (to them, you
cannot be Black and gay) or because they feel they will be ex-
cluded from the African American community if they label
themselves "gay." Many also feel that the term "gay" is so identified with Whites that it does not include them. In order to convey information about safe sex, educators coined a new term,
MSM, to try to reach this "hidden" population.

African American lesbians, meanwhile, have to combat three
strikes against them in U.S. society: being Black, female and lesbian, all of which makes them targets for harassment and discrimination, and all of which present unique challenges. A
seventeen-year-old African American lesbian who grew up in
Harlem and is a first-generation American (her family came from
Jamaica) describes her mindset before she came to terms with
her homosexuality: "I had to get rid of my own internal homophobia and a lifetime of anti-homosexual programming. Growing up, I had feelings for other women. I didn't know what they
meant, but I knew I was taught it was not right, and I hated myself for it. I thought I was the most disgusting thing on the face of
the earth, not worthy of being loved or even existing. . . . I was
ashamed of my background and terrified that someone might
find out that I was a lesbian."

The need to create an ethnic community as a safe place,
driven by the reality of living in a racist society, has made community very important to many African Americans. The Christian church has often been the bedrock of that community, with

unfortunate consequences for LGBTQ people in places where those churches have been vocally hostile to LGBTQ people. Many African American parents have taught their children that this community is the only reliable source of support in a hostile society.

Furthermore, they are often told that their role is to perpetuate that community and improve it through a personal example of "good conduct" and adherence to the community's expectations. For many LGBTQ African American youth, this creates a painful dilemma, because they feel they have to choose between their community and their sexual identity, which is rarely commended as a way of "uplifting" the race.

One of the things you can help your child understand is that you can be both Black and LGBTQ. They are not in conflict. They can be integrated successfully.

That concept may be a stretch for you, too. If you believe that homosexuality and doing the right thing by the race are mutually exclusive, as I'm sure many African American parents do, I ask you to try to put aside your beliefs for now. I am not asking you to change them or abandon them, but to support your child.

Latino/a Cultures

Many Latino/a cultures, an umbrella term encompassing (among other groups) Puerto Rican Americans, Mexican Americans, and Chicano/a Americans, honor the following two values:

1. The dominant role of the Catholic Church and its beliefs

2. Highly defined gender roles, i.e., the "machismo" and "marianismo" divide where men are strong and women passive

In Latino/a cultures, the traditional Catholic belief is that the only appropriate sex is sex within the covenant of marriage for the purpose of procreation. Even though virtually no straight people abide by this definition of appropriate sexual relations, it is still held up the chastise LGBTQ people. In this theology, LGBTQ people are simply expected to be celibate for life in order to avoid sin. Catholicism also feeds into traditional Latino/a cultural values concerning gender roles, in which men are supposed to be dominant and macho, and women are passive and forbearing in the manner of the Virgin Mary (known as marianismo).

In this way of thinking any woman who deviates from the Madonna icon—and that includes lesbians—risks social ostracism. Latinas are often discouraged from discussing sex, acknowledging their bodies and seeking pleasure. They are expected to attach to a man and cater to his needs. A Latina lesbian—who enjoys her body, seeks sexual pleasure and doesn't need a man to complete her—is considered an insult to women who accept the conventional arrangement and a traitor to the community. Sometimes, Latinas feel that they can keep their place in the family and the community only if they hide their lesbian identity.

It is not uncommon for Latinos to engage in same-gender sexual behavior, yet like their male African American counterparts, they would never think of calling themselves gay. Being gay is equated with being feminine, and being feminine is not valued in the macho Latino culture. On the other hand, it has sometimes been acceptable to be the dominant partner in a gay sexual relationship if you are a Latino man, as the only person considered "gay" is the receptive partner. This has enabled many Latinos to participate in same-sex sexual behavior without risking a label that might compromise their membership in the community.

For all these reasons, people who are LGBTQ often remain closeted to avoid the ostracism that would result. Some, who do come out, may be quietly tolerated, but that doesn't mean they're accepted. One young man, in frustration, explained his mother's denial of his homosexuality, her encouragement that he have sex with a female friend and her insistence that he keep his sexuality a secret from his younger siblings. Another said, "Unless I bring home grandchildren, I'll never win Mom's approval."

Asian Pacific American Cultures

In Asian Pacific American cultures, including Southeast Asian Pacific Americans, South Asian Pacific Americans, Pacific Americans and Americans of Japanese, Korean and Chinese ancestry, the following characteristics are often prominent:

1. Youths are expected to be obedient to their parents, conform to their wishes, and respect their elders.

2. Life paths are sharply prescribed, based on biological gender.

3. The importance of "face" makes sex a taboo topic that is considered shameful if discussed openly.

In many Asian Pacific American communities, the family is held in the highest regard as the fundamental building block of the community. Family roles are shaped by gender and age. Men are expected to continue the family line and name by marrying and having children. Women have three prescribed roles: First, they are someone's daughter, then someone's wife and then someone's mother. Children often learn from an early age that their obligation is to obey their parents, follow the paths their parents have laid out, and never embarrass the family by publicly deviating from them.

If a child comes out as LGBTQ, he is not only rejecting the traditional role and the importance of family, but he is showing the community that his parents, especially his mother, have failed. Parents often feel ashamed if their neighbors or friends know their child is LGBTQ. One Asian Pacific American mother explained her response to her daughter's coming out: "I told her we would have to move away from this house. I felt strongly that neighbors and friends in the community would not want to associate with us if they knew we had a child who had chosen to be homosexual."

Gay men are seen as disloyal to their tradition and threatening to the family continuity. Similarly, some families may be troubled by having a lesbian daughter who defies the "three roles" laid out for her. LGBTQ Asian Pacific American youth who come out therefore often feel they're in a double bind: They are not only engaging in a behavior that is counter-cultural and shameful, but they are talking about it, which is something you don't do in most Asian Pacific American cultures—no matter what the problem. Public appearance and saving face are critical. By talking about "problems" like being LGBTQ in public, these children bring shame on the family. Being LGBTQ is "bad enough"; talking about it is unacceptable.

Like the young man whose quote opened this chapter, many Asian Pacific American youth feel alienated from their communities because they fear these communities can neither recognize them nor honor them. They often feel they must therefore choose one identity over the other. Often, their inability to reconcile their sexual identity with their culture's traditional ideas about homosexuality lead them to leave their ethnic communities behind. One study found that most Asian Pacific American LGBTQ people identified first as LGBTQ, rather than as Asian Pacific American.

CHOOSING THE "GAY LIFESTYLE"

In all of these cultures of color, there are parents who just can't understand why their child has to be so obvious about his sexual orientation. Why does their son have to live with another man or their daughter with another woman? And more important, why does he have to talk about what he's doing? Why can't he "do his own thing" in private, as generations before have done, rather than choosing the so-called "gay lifestyle"?

The "gay lifestyle" of popular culture is a concept not shared by all LGBTQ people. As many understand it, though, it includes the following two aspects:

1. being open about same-sex orientation and talking about it

2. living outside of heterosexual marriage, often in a same-sex relationship

Traditionally, LGBTQ people of color have not dealt with their sexual orientation in the way that today's largely White LGBTQ culture encourages them to. That is, by speaking openly about their sexual orientation and living outside traditional heterosexual marriage. This explains why some perceive being LGBTQ as a White thing, and to a certain extent it is. The norms associated with the "gay lifestyle" in common usage are those largely of White LGBTQ people, who are the most visible members of the community in the media and in national LGBTQ organizations. The way the "gay lifestyle" is seen in much of America now is largely an outgrowth of this popular image, dominated by White people.

Communities of color have always had and known about the LGBTQ people in their midst, but have not always talked openly about them or felt comfortable with their living outside traditional marital or gender roles. There is a huge difference between knowing that there are LBGTQ people in the community and tolerating them on some level, and accepting the decision of your child to live the modern "gay lifestyle" of open acknowledgment and same-sex partnerships.

Your accepting this decision is so important to your child because it shows that you accept him. Every child, no matter his age or orientation, needs that validation from his parents. It says to him, "You're OK. I love you just the way you are."

Some parents of color may feel that their child is rejecting the "traditional" expectations around family living arrangements in their culture, and he, in fact, may be. But he does not want to reject every aspect of your culture. He simply wants to live his life openly. The choice he is making is not around his sexual orientation, but in how he chooses to express it.

He is not choosing to be LGBT: he is choosing to be honest and authentic.

He is coping with his orientation in a way that may be alien to you. But remember: he is coping with it in a way that is authentic for him. As I've emphasized before, whether your child is Black or White, LGBTQ or straight, the most important requirement for developing into an emotionally healthy adult is to live an authentic life. Any time you have to hide or keep a secret, that produces isolation. Isolated teens are more at risk for problems, as I've stressed throughout this book.

The following quote from a young male high school student of Indian descent will give you an inkling of the torment teens experience when they can't be authentic in their own homes. "I've become so good at passing as straight, it's scary. But it's not a good thing because I know that I'm not being myself. Most of the time, I feel like a prisoner in my own body. I feel like everyone else owns me. 'Being yourself' is much harder done than said. Most of the time, I feel physically uncomfortable. I'm constantly aware of the way my head is tilted, where my hands fall, how my legs are positioned, my facial expression. It's so exhausting. The only place I feel free is when I'm in my room, alone."

He continues, thinking aloud: "If I were 'flaming' around Dad and my brother, they wouldn't exactly appreciate it. And Mom, who knows that I'm gay, wouldn't want me to 'advertise' my sexuality because others in the Indian American community might find out, and what other people think is so damn important to my parents' generation."

ACCEPTING YOUR CHILD

In Chapter 5, I discussed the typical process a parent goes through in coming to accept the fact that she has an LGBTQ child. I explained how each parent has her own process within the general framework I put forth. Please review that chapter now to familiarize yourself with the stages.

The process you are experiencing is similar to every parent's process. Because of your cultural traditions, however, your process may be different in the following three ways:

1. Your stages may be influenced by your cultural back-ground and may trigger many different emotions be-cause of your heritage.

   For example, if you are a Chinese American parent, you may feel ashamed, embarrassed and disappointed if your daughter comes out as a lesbian because she is de-fying the traditional three roles Chinese women play in your culture: those of daughter, wife and mother.

   You must also contend with family expectations that a typical White family does not have. Your first reaction may be: "I know that my mother is expecting Amy to have the same kind of life that she and I have had. She's going to be so ashamed by Amy's coming out and feel it is a great dishonor to our family. How do I explain to her that the same pattern that we've repeated in our family for generations, which we've been told is the only pat-tern that is acceptable for women like us—even women who are lawyers—isn't going to happen for Amy?"

   To figure out how to respond to your mother, I would

again suggest you go back to Chapter 5, the section about telling family members. If you're a first-generation immigrant talking to your mother back in Ecuador or Hong Kong or if you're a second-generation immigrant and your mother is here but still has many "old world" ways, you may need to add something such as the following when you speak to her, "I know this is difficult for you because this is not the way gay people have typically behaved in our culture. But this is how it's done in the United States. We have to try and understand and support Amy as she does things her way, which is going to be different from ours."

Keep in mind that one of the most difficult things for second-generation parents is melding their culture and the American culture, so it may take time for you to see any movement in this area.

2. You may blame yourself for this "problem." If you are a first- or second-generation American, you might castigate yourself, wondering: Why did I move my family here? Maybe I made a mistake. I've exposed them to all these bad influences. Now what they are doing is wrong. I made a bad decision in moving to the United States in the first place.

Keep in mind that LGBTQ teens exist in your home country and your home cultures as well. What is happening here is that your child has adapted to the different way today's U.S. culture typically handles homosexuality.

You probably have had life experiences which mirror this. Today's African American teens have parents who were once "Black" and grandparents who were "Negroes" and great-grandparents who were "colored." Our racial identities evolve over time, and the same is true for sexual identities. The world is different for LGBTQ

African American men today than it was fifty years ago when they might have felt the only choice was to be the church organist and be silent about being LGBT. Your child is not making the wrong choice. He is making choices in a different set of historical circumstances from those you grew up in and that's okay. You've done the same thing yourself.

3. You may feel trapped in the middle between two generations. Your parents and your child are pulling you in opposite directions. You want to be supportive of your child, but at the same time, you may be entrenched in your culture's "traditions" and what they tell you about how LGBTQ people should behave.

You may not realize it, but your child is probably experiencing similar conflicts around his decision to come out. You may feel more compassion for your child if you reflect on the complex process your teenager is going through in trying to integrate all the different parts of his identity. Whatever you are experiencing, your child is probably going through it more intensely. You can use the understanding this generates as a chance to talk openly together and build a new relationship in which you help each other find a way to make this journey successfully. The section on "How You Can Help" starting on page 230 will tell you how to do this.

INTEGRATING AN IDENTITY

There are a lot of stresses on teenagers today. As I remarked earlier in the book, it's tough to figure out gender roles today: how to be a man or a woman in our society. But those concerns are especially magnified when youth come from cultures of color, as the following young man of Indian descent explains: "In progressive circles and classes, we talk about gender norms, and what it means to 'be a man' or 'act like a lady.' I feel the sting of narrow gender norms right now. For years, I've adored the classical Indian dance called Bharatanatyam. It's typically learned and performed by females. But I've always wanted to learn it. So I enrolled in a class with a male instructor a week ago.

"Although the classes are great and I'm happy I signed up, the fact that I have to keep it concealed from my parents is absurd. It's so ridiculous that I have to sneak behind my parents' backs to learn my own culture because of some stupid gender norms. I can just hear my parents: 'It's for girls,' 'What will other people think,' 'Men don't do that.' "

He concludes, "Sometimes I just think it'd be easier for me to have been born a female. I really believe that if that were the case, I wouldn't be so stilted in the way I talk and walk, I could do what I want to do, and I'd be able to laugh and talk freely."

If you're a person of color, your race and ethnicity often form an important part of your identity: who you are. From a young age, you look in the mirror and see that you're Black or yellow or brown, and start thinking about what this means for you in a society that has traditionally accorded its privileges mainly to White people. In most cases, your family looks like you and can help you figure this out. But then, as you approach adolescence (or sometimes younger), you realize that you're attracted to people of the same gender. But what you learned about your cultural "traditions" tells you that this kind of person and this kind of behavior is not acceptable. If it's done at all, it must be done in secret and not talked about.

Consequently, many youth of color feel conflicted and confused as they try to navigate the development of a racial identity as well as a healthy sexual identity. The task of sexual identity development alone is complex for anyone, but it is more complicated for those who are also facing racial identity development issues.

Here is the position your child is in: Just as he's trying to sort out his racial identity, another identity, a sexual or gender one, surfaces that you or your family or community (or all of these) may see as profoundly in conflict with his racial identity.

Your child is thinking: Okay, in my culture the way in which sexual orientation and gender identity issues have been dealt with is not the way broader U.S. culture deals with them, so am I really Black anymore? Am I really Chinese? Am I really Latino?

And you, as a parent, may wonder the same thing: What happened to my child? Is he still Asian/Black/Latino?

To a LGBTQ teen of color, the decision to come out can feel like a double betrayal: He's deviating from your family and your cultural communities. For some teens, this is simply too much to deal with. A young man from Iowa explains, "A lot of youth of color are simply not dealing with their sexual orientations. Many people of color have been told their whole life: 'You're a racial minority, this is your obstacle and you just kind of have to deal with it.' So when it comes time to deal with sexual orientation, they follow this mindset of 'This is my issue and I need to deal with it on my own, without being vocal.' "

Young LGBTQ people also feel torn because the institutions for people of color are often not welcoming to LGBTQ people and the institutions of the LGBTQ community, which are largely White, are not welcoming to people of color. So youth feel conflicted: Is it possible to be both Black and gay? Where do I truly belong? Whenever you put a young person in a situation where he has to choose among identities or give up part of who he is, that is a recipe for disaster.

Trying to deny part of yourself is an exhausting and demoralizing experience. Having to lie and hide every day can lead to depression, self-hatred and self-destructive behavior, as earlier chapters in the book have made all too clear. The chances of being forced to do so are more likely for LGBTQ youth of color, and thus they can be at especially high risk.

Your child is navigating totally new terrain on his own, and needs nothing more than your unconditional understanding.

HOW YOU CAN HELP

Your most important task is to help your child develop a healthy racial identity and a healthy sexual identity that are not in opposition to each other. Just as there is not just one way to experience homophobia, and not just one way to become and be LGBTQ, there is not just one way for you to support your child.

Here are seven ways that have worked for other parents of color. As you read these suggestions, keep in mind that just because you support your LGBTQ child, it doesn't mean that you are rejecting your own culture.

But you must support your child: His life is at stake.

1. Think about how you resolved conflicts with your parents about ideas and practices related to your racial identity. You probably don't understand or express your Blackness, Asian-ness or Latino-ness in the same way your parents did. Perhaps you were the first African American person to go to college in your family. Remember when education was perceived as "White" by some African American people? Or maybe your children grew up speaking English instead of Spanish, as you did.

   In each of these cases—and you can probably think of other examples—you have already undergone some identity evolution of your own in which you've had to explain to your parents or grandparents that you are still just as Black or Asian Pacific or Latino as they, even though the way in which you express your racial identity is not the same as the way they did.

   While this subject matter (homosexuality) may at first

seem strange and foreign to you, you've been through this *process* before. If you're an immigrant, for instance, you've already had to find a way to mix your home country's culture with that of America in a way that works for you. Your job now is to apply those skills to a different challenge for your child.

Remember: You know how to do this. You've done it before.

2. Share the information you learned about yourself with your LGBTQ child. You can say to him, "Even though I'm not LGBTQ and haven't experienced what you're going through, I have had to face similar issues with my parents." Then relate the particular issue that was problematic for you and your parents. For example, you might say something such as, "You know grandpa only went through sixth grade. I went to Boston University. That doesn't make me any less African American than he is, but he had a hard time because he thought I was deserting the race by going to a 'White' institution.

"He wanted me to go to Spelman and he was afraid somehow I would lose touch with being Black by going to a 'White' college. But I found that you can be just as 'Black' as anybody else, even if the path you're taking is different from that taken by previous generations of our family. Just because the way you're expressing yourself as a gay, Black person is different from me—your straight, Black parent—it doesn't mean that you aren't Black anymore."

3. Remind your child that LGBT people of color have always existed in our society and always will. Point out role models in our culture of LGBTQ people of color who have successfully integrated their racial and sexual identities. Mention people like the writer Alice Walker, the comedian Margaret Cho, and Massachusetts State

Representative Jarret Barrios, who have all been open about their same-sex relationships and are still seen as "authentically" African American, Korean American, and Latino, respectively.

4. Give your child examples of other people who have found ways to create authentic racial identities for themselves while engaging in professions, behaviors or lifestyles that do not conform to what their ethnic community has traditionally done. I'm not talking about LGBTQ role models but about the broad variety of people from each cultural group that exists in society who have found ways to integrate things that are seemingly foreign. Think of Leontyne Price and Jessye Norman, African American singers who have conquered that "Whitest" of all musical genres, opera (and in Norman's case, done it while also singing African American spirituals at Lincoln Center).

5. Recognize that "cultural traditions" aren't written in stone, and can, do and should evolve.

Those who loudly proclaim that LGBTQ people are "foreign" to their culture's "traditions" often don't even have their facts "straight" (to use a little pun). For example, a Native American who says that LGBTQ people "don't belong" in native communities must have forgotten that the Zuni people sent a Two Spirit (a man who lived as a woman) named We'wha as their ambassador to Washington in the 1880s. The negative feelings this person has toward transgendered people would mystify his ancestors, who venerated and esteemed such people.

Culture is what we make of it and is always evolving. As we all move through life, we develop in our understanding of our cultures, discarding some beliefs as outdated, acquiring new perceptions, and ending up in very different places from where we, our parents and our ancestors started. That's a positive thing, as we all need to find a way to adapt our cultures to changing times.

In this case, a little evolution would probably do you and your family—and certainly your LGBTQ child—a little good. Don't be afraid to change: people always have.

6. Help your child come out to other family members so he doesn't have to bear that burden alone. In Chapter 5, I discussed ways to broach the subject with other family members. Review that chapter now and then discuss with your child whom he will tell, when he will tell them and how he will break the news. Offer to be present with him or to be the bearer of the news, if he prefers and you are comfortable with that role.

7. Find support for your child. There are three kinds of support that can help ease the isolation your child is probably feeling:

• Try to locate other LGBTQ youth of your ethnic heritage. This may be difficult unless you live in a large city. Here are three ways to get started:

1. Go to the gay-straight alliance in your child's high school.

2. Ask at a PFLAG meeting.

3. Look for local groups specific to your ethnic background through the national web sites listed in the Resources section at the back of the book.

If you have any doubts about why this is so important, listen to the words of a Cambodian lesbian who felt completely isolated until she discovered another Cambodian lesbian: "It's important for me to feel that

I'm not a freak. Yeah, there are Korean lesbians, there are Chinese lesbians, etc. But there aren't any Cambodian lesbians. I met one just a couple of months ago and I felt so good. I was in tears almost, because it was like looking at myself in the mirror. I'm not alone."

Finding such support for your child is invaluable. Yet you may feel that I'm asking you to do a lot or too much. Keep in mind that young people of color need extra support so they can meet other young people like themselves. This is not easy, as many GSAs or PFLAG chapters are often largely, if not wholly, White. If you don't feel you can do this yourself, encourage your child to do so and keep checking in to see how he's doing.

• Read books to find how others have successfully integrated their racial and sexual identities. You can do this in the following three ways:

1. Check out the list of recommended books in the Resources section at the back of this book for suggestions.

2. Go to your local bookstore and browse the Gender Studies section.

3. Ask other parents to recommend books that have been helpful to them when you meet them at a PFLAG meeting.

• Find web sites geared to LBGTQ individuals of your particular ethnic group. Several are listed at the Resources section at the back of this book.

COMING TO TERMS

Your child is not going to live his life by the same script that you did. He is not going to follow your generation's ideas about sexual identity and racial identity—just as you didn't want to live out your parents' script. Your child has his own life to live. By supporting him in figuring out his own process in the ways we've discussed in this chapter, your acceptance and love will help give him the confidence and courage to live an authentic life.

I know this may not be easy for you. But remember, you are not alone either. Other parents have faced similar struggles. I hope Belinda Rayos Del Sol Dronkers-Laureta's* story will give you the strength and courage to be there for your son or daughter.

Belinda was born in the Philippines and came to America when she was ten. Until the age of nineteen, she lived in a Filipino American community in California. She has a large extended family, both in the states and in the Philippines. As an adult, she married, bought a house, and raised three children. She worked her entire life to make the American dream a reality and hoped her children would do the same.

In 1993, she received a phone call from her second child, Lance, that changed her life. Lance is a gifted child who received a scholarship to Sarah Lawrence to study cinematography. Today, he is a youth educator for the Grant Street Settlement Project in Queens, New York. Prior to that, he was youth coordinator for the Asian Pacific Islander Coalition HIV Association (APICHA).

Out of the blue, Lance told her he had been to Washington D.C. to march in the Gay Pride Parade.

"Does that mean you are gay?" she asked.

"Yes," he replied.

---

* This story is adapted from an article in the November 23, 2001 issue of *AsianWeek*.

Belinda explains her reaction, "I didn't have the slightest idea what it meant to be gay or the implications of having a gay son. Not just then. But I do remember that during that telephone conversation, a numbness came over me; a strange feeling of being in one place, but at the same time being far away; of talking to my middle child, yet talking to a stranger."

After she talked with Lance she called her husband at work and told him their son was a homosexual. He didn't "get" it either.

She continues, "The first two years after Lance told me his secret were terrible. My thoughts and emotions were all mixed up. At first, I hoped it was just a phase he was going through—you know how teenagers are. But it wasn't. I was also disappointed that I would have no daughter-in-law or grandchildren to visit.

"At the time, with no knowledge and little support, I couldn't help but feel like he was being stupid and selfish with his 'homosexual' attitude. I was afraid for his safety. I was afraid of people who hate homosexuals: they jeer, they call the police, they throw stones, they attack.

"I worried that Lance wouldn't find peace anywhere and that he would have to flee all the time. I was ashamed. I thought of my son as being one of those gay people who do unnatural things. My family and friends would find out. They would think that I raised a Bakla or Binabae—a man who acts like a female. In the Philippines, homosexuals are looked upon as bad people. They don't belong anywhere. There isn't even a word for 'gay' in Tagalog. The words are all derogatory. I cried a lot during those two years."

But gradually, over that two-year period, Belinda came to realize, "This was my son. I gave birth to him. He was not weird. He could not be bad. I raised him and he is so talented."

All along Belinda knew that she did not want to lose her child. She never thought of disowning him although she worried that their community would isolate him. She explains, "I had to get educated. I had to understand why some people are gay and what it means."

Her husband and the two other children helped. Lance sent pamphlets from PFLAG. He answered her many questions. At her husband's work, the gay and lesbian employee association organized an information panel. She went and asked many questions there, too. She went to the library and bookstores to read and learn.

On Father's Day in 1995, two years after her son came out, Belinda, her husband, and daughter marched in the San Francisco Gay Pride Parade. There she met people who have LGBT children with whom she could talk about being a parent to a gay son.

After a while, she was able to mention to people outside her family that she has a gay son. She says, "I began telling close friends, then acquaintances, and then everybody who asked why Lance wasn't married yet."

In March 1996, she co-founded the Fremont, California, chapter of PFLAG and one month later she became its president and attended both regional and national meetings. She joined organizations in the San Francisco Bay Area to help Asian and Pacific Islander parents accept and understand their LGBT children.

PFLAG's San Francisco Chapter supported the Asian/Pacific Islander Family Project. That has now spun off into an independent organization called API Family Pride. She and her husband are members of the board.

Recently she said, "I look upon that April 1993 phone call as an event that changed my life. I didn't know it then, but that day began a journey, and a fabulous journey it has been. I met great people, made many new friends, but most of all, I am closer to my children than ever before. Especially, I am close to Lance and I am so proud of him. He taught me so much.

"No one should be isolated and no one has the right to isolate."

Chapter Nine

OUTSIDE THE HOME

Advocating for Your LGBTQ Teen at School

AS THE YOUNGEST of four athletic boys, I loved sports, but I did not like my gym class. I tried to steer clear of my teacher Mr. Hooker because he seemed to have a smoldering rage. But there were even greater problems.

Sometime in the winter of seventh grade we did a unit on wrestling. I began to approach class with dread, as I feared for my ability to keep my feelings successfully hidden from my largely fundamentalist classmates. Gary was the most distracting of all. With feathered blond hair parted in the middle and a firm muscular body, he entranced me, even though I hated him and, more important, myself because I could barely take my eyes off him.

I was fighting this internal battle on the day we began the wrestling unit. As Mr. Hooker went on about the sport's scoring system, I couldn't take my eyes away from Gary, who was blissfully absorbed in Mr. Hooker's lecture. Mr. Hooker, however, seemed more attuned to where my eyes were focused. He stopped in mid-sentence, fixed his gaze on me, and very slowly and clearly said, "Stop looking at his legs."

As my classmates slowly turned to look at me amidst the dead silence in the wrestling room, I felt as if a stake had been driven through my heart. A few moments of silence passed and Mr. Hooker then went back to his lecture.

I never went back to being the person I was before that moment.

I never played on an organized school team again, even though playing sports was (and is) a source of great joy for me.

I never again felt as though I belonged at school.

I never forgot Mr. Hooker.

This experience took place in 1976, over twenty-five years ago. As we saw in Chapter 4, sexism, anti-LGBT bias and harassment are still rampant in schools across the country. Not just among students. Not only do coaches and teachers look the other way and say nothing, but often they are participants. This probably comes as a shock to you, especially if you grew up in a generation that revered teachers.

In this chapter, I'll explore the reasons why school administrators and teachers are often uncomfortable with sexual identity issues, ill-equipped to handle problems, and sometimes even homophobic themselves. I'll offer you practical suggestions for how and when to take action in school issues, how to pinpoint the root of the problem and how to find appropriate solutions. Throughout the chapter, I'll sprinkle groundbreaking decisions that mark the progress LGBT rights activists have made. They are quite graphic and may disturb you, but I hope they will inspire you to protect your child.

Many parents are dangerously out of touch with what really goes on regarding LGBT issues in our schools and how urgent the need for action is. Furthermore, I believe an ounce of prevention is worth a pound of cure. In this chapter we will not only look at how to react if your child is in immediate danger, but how to take preventive action to improve your school, so there is less likelihood that a crisis will ever occur.

DID YOU KNOW?

Teachers, counselors and principals who are unhelpful or hurtful may be violating the law in failing to address anti-LGBT abuse. Such violations may place their licenses in jeopardy. Professional associations in states such as Florida, have adopted codes of conduct that include an expectation that teachers will not discriminate based on sexual orientation. Using these, as well as support from teachers' unions (both the National Education Association and the American Federation of Teachers have clear policies on sexual orientation) can either shame or compel teachers to act more professionally and appropriately.

FACTS FIRST

When peers pick on LGBTQ youth, they turn to the authorities—teachers, coaches, counselors—for protection. When the authority itself is the culprit, students feel devastated, vulnerable and alone.

According to GLSEN's 2001 National School Climate Survey, over 80 percent of youth reported that faculty or staff never intervened or intervened only some of the time when homophobic remarks were made. That means they ignore homophobic remarks and slurs in class or in the hall, look the other way, or turn a deaf ear.

They do not say a word.

That's horrendous in itself. It's quite another thing, however, to be the perpetrators of those comments. According to the same survey, one quarter of youth reported hearing anti-LGBT remarks from faculty or school staff some of the time. I want to share three moving stories with you, so you fully understand the pain that LGBTQ youth experience at the mercy of their teachers and coaches. Keep in mind, though, that these stories could come from any school in America.

• One young girl told me that every day when she came to school, a group of boys would corner her in the hallway at the beginning of school and say, "You little dyke. Some day we are going to f**k you until you turn straight." I was obviously horrified and asked her, "Have you told the authorities about this?" She started laughing. I said, "What's so funny?" She said, "Mr. Jennings, where do you think this school's security guard stands? He stands at that front door. He watches this happen every morning." She was being harassed directly in front of the person who is paid to protect her.

• In Crown Point, Indiana, an eighth-grader's parents are suing his history teacher, accusing the man of giving the boy a candy valentine heart in which he scratched off the printed message on the candy and wrote the word "fag" on it and gave it to the boy in front of his fellow students. The teacher is also accused of pointing a TV remote control at students while pretending it was a "fagometer." The teacher lost his job but, unfortunately, the school district turned down an offer of free resources and training from GLSEN, indicating that they are still in denial about the fact that they have problems.

• David Ortmann hated chemistry because the teacher, Ms. Frico, was always late. While they waited for her, the class told "fag" jokes. One day Joe C. was discussing with Denise, a cheerleader, one of their classmate's sexual orientation. "No, really, Denise, what do you think?" Joe asked.

At that point the Ms. Frico entered. David was relieved. Usually class was a safe haven for him. Unbeknownst to Joe and Denise, Ms. Frico overheard part of their conversation. "Yeah, Denise, what do you think?" she asked as she crossed the room to her desk smiling.

"I dunno," Denise replied.

Then Ms. Frico looked directly at David Ortmann, smiled, and said, "Joe, why don't you just ask Mr. Ortmann. He should know. He's a fag."

For a moment, there was an unbelieving silence and then half the class erupted with kids laughing, pounding their desks and spilling into the aisle. The rest of the class continued to stare, disbelieving. David recalls, "My gut burned. My spine tightened and cracked. My throat immediately went dry. Flushing crimson, beads of sweat broke out on my brow. I dared not move as I felt like I could cry, puke, shit, and piss all at once. I wanted to run. Run home. Run somewhere . . . anywhere but here. But I just sat there unbelieving . . . this is not supposed to happen! A teacher can't say that!"

WHAT'S THEIR PROBLEM?

There is no acceptable explanation for anti-LGBT comments by teachers, but I will try to give you a context for understanding why we have reached this juncture. There are five reasons that account for it:

1. Like everyone else, teachers are human beings. They bring the same kind of baggage into their professional work as everybody else does. Much as we would like to think that all professionals—teachers, doctors etc.— check their prejudices when they put on their professional hat, they just don't.

2. Not all education schools or professional development training programs address LGBT issues. GLSEN did a survey of the forty-two largest school districts in the U.S. in 1998. We found that 76 percent of them had no workshops for teachers to learn about LGBTQ issues. Little seems to have changed in the major dis-

tricts since 1998 and based on anecdotal evidence, the situation is even worse in small towns. So, teachers in training receive no education on LGBTQ concerns and no continuing education training once they're in the profession.

3. The high median age for teachers accounts for some prejudice. A huge number of teachers are going to retire in the next ten to fifteen years, which means they are in their late forties or early fifties. Older teachers tend to be more conservative, and may not personally know LBGTQ people, as younger teachers often do.

4. If teachers stick their necks out, there is no institutional support. Some are afraid that if they intervene, they'll be seen as LGBT. In New York State, for example, there is no law that says a teacher can't be fired for being LGBT. This is true in thirty-seven other states as well. Even if they aren't LGBT, they fear that rumors will spread to that effect and if they come up for tenure, the school board may decide that the rumors may harm their school, so the teacher is denied tenure.

In GLSEN's first round of focus groups in the Chicago suburb of Oak Park on June 14, 2001, teachers told us that the administration would never back them up if they supported LGBT issues. The following story will give you a sense of what it means to have no institutional support: The Sunday magazine of a large metropolitan city newspaper ran a feature about the problems of LGBT high school students. A school principal wanted to write a letter to the editor praising the article, but she felt that if her name appeared in the paper she would jeopardize her job. She agonized over what to do and finally decided to write the letter but asked a friend who was not in the school system to sign her name instead.

5. Discomfort with LGBT issues. Many teachers think

Whenever you can, push for training for teachers in your school district. They desperately need more self-awareness and understanding, so they can become more conscious of how their own prejudices and biases harm students. The way to begin this process is to find an ally on the school board who will set the training in motion.

these issues are so unusual that what they would normally do around harassment would not work. That's just not true. But because LGBTQ issues are so loaded in our culture, many teachers believe they don't have any expertise in this area and don't know what to do. The reality is that because they have received no training or support, they feel threatened themselves, undermined by their administration and its policies, and disempowered by their own lack of familiarity with the issues.

WHAT YOU CAN DO

Your first priority is to make sure that your child is safe physically and feels supported psychologically, so that he can devote his energy to learning. After all, that's why he's in school.

To achieve that, we must all work with those who have the power and responsibility to stop the abuse. That can feel like an overwhelming task. You may not even know where to begin, so I'm going to take you step by step through the process of what to do if your child is the victim of harassment or other inequitable treatment.

Here are the eight steps to follow*:

*The information in this section is adapted from Lambda's brochure, "Stopping Anti-Gay Bias of Students in Public Schools: A Legal Perspective."

1. Determine if your school or state has a policy that protects students based on sexual orientation or gender identity.

   Begin by locating the student handbook. Students are supposed to bring them home to their parents but many don't. The handbook will set forth the school's policies on discrimination. You can get it at the principal's office.

   'To get a copy of the state policies, go to the web sites of GLSEN, the ACLU, or Lambda Legal Defense and Education Fund. They are listed in the Resources section at the back of the book.

   Also consider whether there are other policies that you might be able to use. In the 1998 case of *Wagner v. Fayetteville*, William Wagner brought a sex discrimination complaint against his school district for failing to protect him from years of harassment. The landmark decision established that same-sex, student-on-student sexual harassment could be considered a violation of the Title IX statute that prohibits sex discrimination and sexual harassment—as long as there is an explicit sexual element to the abuse. You cannot apply Title IX if some-

---

DID YOU KNOW?

When right-wing extremists tried to bring the idea of "reparative therapy" to the schools in late 1998, ten prestigious mainstream mental health and education groups, including the American Association of School Administrators, the American Psychological Association and the American Academy of Pediatrics, banded together and published "Just the Facts about Sexual Orientation and Youth" and sent it to every superintendent in the country, telling them that it is our schools, not our youth, who need to be "fixed." You can obtain a copy at GLSEN's web site, www.glsen.org

one says, "You faggot." They have to say, "I'm going to f**k you, you little faggot."

2. Build allies both within and outside the system.

To do this:

- Think of the school-based and community-based resources in your area, including advocacy groups, such as GLSEN, PFLAG, Lambda, ACLU or the Anti-Defamation League. Also consider the Teacher's Union, the Parent Teacher Association and your clergy.
- Call the organization and get the president's name and phone number.
- Explain your situation.
- Ask how the organization can help you or whether they've been involved in similar situations.
- Find out if you can go to the next meeting.

There are two important reasons to build allies:

1. You will have more clout when you have an organization behind you. Many times when parents complain, officials think, "Oh, it's just that crazy parent overreacting again." When you have an organization supporting you, it helps school officials realize that the problem is not limited to just one child or one overreacting parent. By building allies, you reinforce the idea that your child doesn't have the problem. The system does.

2. Retribution from school officials and classmates is a very real problem. Building an emotional support system for you and your child may lessen some of your fears because you will not have to face your detractors alone. You will have an organization behind you.

3. Look into complaint procedures.

Complaint procedures vary greatly. The school's formal complaint procedures may apply to any complaint of student misconduct or they may be very specific and apply to just one type of complaint, such as sexual harassment. They also may be applicable statewide, regionally or just to one particular school.

These procedures are not always easy to locate. You may have to track them down by contacting several individuals to find out which procedures are applicable in your child's case.

Once you know the procedures, you have to figure out what would be the best way to advance your cause. If you find that the procedure for making a formal complaint has too many steps and will take too long, you may want to begin that and also start a parallel process of climbing the ladder to the school board or superintendent.

4. Report the abuse.

Schools cannot take action if they don't know about the abuse. You must tell the principal. Counselors and teachers can be an important part of your support system, but they do not have the same level of authority or legal obligation to take action. Remember to report all forms of abuse, not just physical abuse. Telling the principal can help promote understanding and begin a dialogue, but your words must be backed up by a written document.

DID YOU KNOW?

Teachers, counselors and principals may violate state child abuse statutes if they don't report abuse to the state authorities. Failure to do so can have serious consequences.

School officials may or may not be responsive. But at least if you're complaining, you are bringing attention to a problem. You are not being passive. Taking action sends an important message to your child.

5. Document what happened.

There is also a higher likelihood of stopping abuse when it is in writing. If the matter should go to litigation later on, verbal reports are not as reliable. Without documentation, one person may say, "But I told you twenty times what was going on" and someone else can deny the conversation, saying, "I never knew about it."

In your written complaint, include the following details:

- Describe the problem in detail: where, when and how
- Name the person or people who harassed your child
- Name all the people you've told about the abuse and write down what you said. For example, "I told the principal on September 21. When we talked, he said he would investigate and take action by October 1."
- Identify the most dangerous parts of the abuse and describe them in detail (there may be more than one). They may include:

    name-calling
    yelling
    being held or trapped
    hitting or kicking
    threats
    use of weapons
    being outnumbered
    adults involved
    sexual assaults
    repeated problems

There have been instances in which school officials have denied receiving a written document. Therefore, you should get some form of proof of receipt. The following work well:

- Have the principal's assistant sign and date your copy of the letter.
- Send your letter by certified mail with a return receipt requested.
- Write the following statement and have it notarized: "My name is . . . and on this date . . . , I personally delivered . . . to . . . , the original of the attached copy of . . ."

Do not underestimate the importance of witnesses. It's harder to take action if it's just the abused student's word against that of his assailant. If the witnesses are willing, have them prepare a written, detailed, signed statement about what happened. Do not let that paper out of your sight until you have made copies and put them in a safe place.

When you write the document, try to use a positive tone and stick to the facts. Saying things like "Your school has totally failed to protect my child" is likely to get a defensive response. Instead, give examples of what has actually happened, and that point will be made more clearly and effectively. Give the principal the benefit of the doubt at this point, and he or she is more likely to respond than if you badger him or her.

6. Move up the ladder.

Some principals are homophobic. Some do not take the complaint seriously; they just let it die in a pile of papers on their desk. Others do not respond in an effective manner. Just giving the abuser a "talking-to" is not effective. More appropriate responses include:

- parent conferences combined with detention
- suspension
- at times, expulsion

An inappropriate—but not uncommon—response is to punish the abused student by:

- changing his class schedule
- moving his seat
- suggesting he transfer to another school.

Derek Henkel came out on a local television program while he was a ninth-grader at a high school in Nevada. From that time on, he was targeted with verbal and physical abuse almost every day. In one incident, his attackers repeatedly lassoed a rope around his neck in the school parking lot and threatened to kill him by dragging him from their truck. Instead of ensuring his safety, school authorities transferred him to an alternative school for troubled students, where the principal told him to "stop acting like a fag." After transferring to a third school, he was beaten bloody by another student while two school security guards stood by and watched. At this point, school officials told him to take classes at a community college to obtain a GED.

This disturbing example shows how school officials can blame the victim for the abuse and let the abuser get off.

Because principals do not always act appropriately, it is sometimes necessary to climb the ladder above their office. Usually the superintendent of the school district or the school board is the next step on the ladder, although the lines of authority may differ from place to place. The state's education department is often beyond the superintendent.

To take your complaint beyond the principal:

- Make an appointment with the person directly above the principal and bring a copy of the written documents.

- Tell the authority what happened.
- Suggest what you would like done to remedy the situation. (Solutions will be explored later in the chapter.)

If you have not built allies, as I suggested earlier, now is the time to do it. This will increase attention to the problem and highlight the school's failure to remedy the situation.

7. Look beyond complaint letters.

If all else fails, there are legal remedies. See the Appendix for details on how to proceed with a lawsuit.

There is no way of knowing what legal possibilities are available until a lawyer looks at the particular facts of the case and consults the laws of your jurisdiction. It is very important, should a lawsuit result, to keep a written record or list of abusive or unfair treatment, including names and dates.

Also look for other avenues of support. For example, if you find that when a boy hits his girlfriend, he is suspended but if he hits a lesbian, nothing is done, then you may have a case under "equal protection" principles. These principles are spelled out in the Fourteenth Amendment of the Constitution, which says that all people are entitled to equal protection under its laws. If you can show that laws are not being applied equally to protect LGBT students, you may have an equal protection case.

Stay attuned to other "leaks" in the system. For example, if a principal is quoted in a local newspaper as saying that a student should expect problems if he is openly LGBT, that quotation could be relevant evidence if a lawyer is trying to prove that the principal was indifferent to your complaints.

Keep documents of any related items such as damning newspaper articles against the principal or a hate note passed to your child that may further support the unfairness of the situation.

8. Be ready with solutions.

We always hope that a principal or administrator will be responsive to complaints but they don't always know what to do, other than to punish the offender. You can help guide them in this by approaching them with specific suggestions of what you want them to do. The following two sections will direct you on how to proceed.

> **TIP:** For information on how to propose changes, go to GLSEN's web site, www.glsen.org, and look at The GLSEN Workbook, which provides a comprehensive assessment tool for helping schools understand how to improve LGBTQ issues.

FINDING SOLUTIONS

> ### CHECKLIST
> As you accomplish each of the above tasks, check them off in the list that follows:
>
> _____ Get safe first
> _____ Report abuse to the school principal
> _____ Document the abuse
> _____ Move up the ladder
> _____ Look into complaint procedures
> _____ Move beyond complaint letters
> _____ Be ready with solutions

Once you identify the specific issue on which you will focus, you have several options about how to solve the problem. Talk with your child about them by saying, "Here is where I see the problem, and here are some responses. What do you think? Let's discuss the best way to proceed."

Whatever the outcome, your actions will teach your child an important lesson: that there are options for problems. The situation is not hopeless. There is always a route to empowerment.

If you want to be helpful in your child's school, at the very least you must insist that policies, such as antiharassment and anti-discrimination are in place, that teachers are trained to deal with the issues, and that the curriculum reflects the real world. While these policies don't always end homophobia, they help to create a more tolerant culture.

In many states, for example, sexuality education classes only teach abstinence until marriage. That is not the reality for a lot of teens. They are not going to abstain until marriage and offering a sexuality curriculum that says that is the only appropriate behavior is not meeting their needs.

Library collections, too, should represent the entire student body. In December 2000, two junior high school students in Orange County, California, filed a federal lawsuit for the right to have biographies of people who are LGBT in their school library. Backed by the American Civil Liberties Union of Southern California, the students demanded that the district return ten books in the series Lives of Notable Gay Men and Lesbians that had "disappeared" from their Orangeview Junior High School Library.

Below I've illustrated three common problems that LGBTQ youth experience and several approaches for solving them. Consider which of the options below would be appropriate for the situation at your child's school:

1. Anti-LGBT name-calling and harassment
   - Pass nondiscrimination and antiharassment policies inclusive of sexual orientation and gender identity.
   - Institute mandatory staff training on responding to name-calling and harassment.

- Implement lesson plans that sensitize students to problems about anti-LGBT bias.
2. No support services for LGBTQ youth
    - Institute training for guidance staff on LGBTQ issues.
    - Create a district position focused on LGBTQ health issues.
    - Raise or commit funds to contract outside agencies to provide services to LGBTQ youth.
3. Invisibility of LGBT people and themes in the curriculum
    - Pass a multicultural or diversity policy that mandates including LGBT themes in the curriculim.
    - Hold staff trainings on integrating LGBT themes into the curriculum.
    - Adopt inclusive texts and other school materials.

> **TIP:** For a more comprehensive and in-depth, systematic approach to solving these kinds of problems, consult The GLSEN Workbook at our web site, www.glsen.org

GUIDELINES FOR MAKING CHANGES

Education and agitation are often lengthy processes before change happens. Some of these general guidelines may work in your situation; others may not. Every situation is unique, depending on the following three factors:

1. the particular school, the climate at the school and in the community

> ### DID YOU KNOW?
> Only thirteen states include the topic of sexual orientation anywhere in their curricula, according to a survey by the Sexuality Information and Education Council of the U.S. (SIECUS).

2. the hierarchy involved

3. the approach you and your allies take.

To change or institute a school policy, following these three steps:

1. Approach the local school board or perhaps even state legislators to convince them to enact changes.

2. Present model policies to show them.

3. Line up organizational allies who can support you.

To change or add new programs, such as teacher training, start with the superintendent or the principal. These folks determine what kinds of training are offered to teachers, help direct curricular and extracurricular program content, and insure that policies are enforced. They also set the tone and are crucial leaders in any change effort.

DID YOU KNOW?

If a school receives federal funding and has non-curricular school clubs, as most do, a gay-straight alliance is entitled to recognition just like any other student group under the federal law called the Equal Access Act.

To improve practices in the school, the following people in the schools are critical here:

- Principals can make public statements encouraging respect for all.
- Teachers can intervene when anti-LGBT language is used and diversify the materials they use in their classes.

- Professionals such as librarians can broaden the materials they offer to students.
- Students can organize gay-straight alliances and lead the process of educating their peers.

A school culture can change when appropriate policies are in place and when administrators offer training and other programatic support, but never forget that an individual administrator, educator or student can still make a difference—even when the rest of the system refuses to "do the right thing."

"BUT I'M NOT AN ACTIVIST"

Your first concern is always your child's safety and that may be your only concern. Some parents just want to get the bully suspended or the teacher in question fired.

That's fine, but in most cases, getting rid of a bully or firing a teacher does not eliminate the problem. They usually act out because they're in a climate that enables them to do so. In the hundreds of schools I've visited, I've learned that when there's one bully, there are usually more. It is rare that there is just one bad apple. If you get rid of the bad apple and another one surfaces and you complain again, then you get labeled as that crazy overreacting parent complaining again. You are less likely to get results.

Many parents do not see themselves as activists, but as they get more involved in trying to protect their child, they are drawn into activist work. They become activists because that's the only way they can get better treatment for their child.

IF YOUR CHILD DOESN'T WANT YOU
TO TAKE AN ACTIVIST ROLE

There are two ways that parents learn about harassment: either from their child or on their own. If your child approaches you, he obviously wants you to step forward. That's one of the reasons he's telling you. It's very rare that a child has revealed what's happening to a parent and then says, "I don't want you to do anything."

The real problem is that, because of shame and embarrassment, youth don't always tell their parents when they are being harassed. When the parent finds out about an act of harassment from a source other than their child and then the child realizes the parent is going to go do something, the child can panic.

If you find out on your own, you still have to go to your child and say, "This is what I want to do. Let's see how we can work together." You need to set that baseline, because your child hasn't approached you for one or more of the following three reasons:

1. He doesn't think you are going to be supportive.

2. He doesn't think you have an ability to make a difference.

3. He's terrified that anything you do is going to bring further abuse.

When I say establish a baseline, I mean making it clear to your child that you have to do something. I suggest you say to him, "Look, standing by and watching this happen and doing nothing is just not acceptable. That's not even on the table for discussion. We can discuss the options we can follow. We can discuss what we're going to do—but not *whether* we do anything."

Make sure that he understands that certain things are non-negotiable. You can say, "I cannot let the authorities *not* do their job. One of my roles as a parent is to make sure that you're safe. You can't learn in a hostile environment." You can also say, "I pay taxes in this school district. I send you there every day and I've got rights too."

Then listen to his objections. Make sure he knows that you hear him. You can respond by saying, "I hear you" or "I see" but then repeat the reasons you gave him before so he understands why this is nonnegotiable. Some youth repeatedly question their parents to test how serious their parent is about taking action. Repeated questioning may not reflect fear or reluctance as much as it reflects conscious or unconscious doubt that you are really going to fight for your LGBTQ child.

After all, these youth often have seen little to lead them to believe that you will, and may want "proof." Hang in there and make it clear you're going to stand by their side and fight hard for them.

Part of what you are communicating is the sense that there is a baseline level of human dignity, which you will not allow to be compromised, to which you are legally entitled and to which authorities have to be held accountable.

That is a very important message for young people to hear. When they have stood by and seen the authorities do nothing, it's utterly demoralizing and contributes to their feeling of worthlessness. You are teaching your child—not so much about being LGBT but how democracy works, that we can stand up for ourselves and we don't have to endure second-rate behavior.

And, that you care about his well-being.

It's also important to acknowledge to your child as you go through this process, "Look, I might not be able to get you what you want. We're going to do our best here. We are going to be in this together, and I'm going to be there for you. I promise I am going to get you to a safe place. If that means I have to take you out of this school, I'll do it."

STRENGTH IN NUMBERS

Advocating for your child can challenge even the most determined parent. Of course, I hope you accomplish everything you set out to achieve. But even if you don't, you are teaching your child three important lessons:

1. the importance of talking about problems in a civil way

2. the value of standing up for himself

3. the need to enlist support

You don't have to do this alone. The organizations we discussed in this chapter are your allies; they have had experience with situations like yours and have resources to draw on. In addition, familiarize yourself with videotapes on homophobia and organizations that provide speakers and trainers for schools and educators. See the Resources section at the back of this book for details on what services and resources each organization offers and for additional suggestions.

Chapter Ten

DEPRESSION, DRUG ABUSE AND SUICIDE

Recognizing Signs of Trouble

ONE DAY WHEN I was teaching at Concord Academy in Massachusetts, I received a phone call from "Jennifer," a young woman who was struggling to come to terms with her sexual orientation. She was one of the heads of our gay-straight alliance and had taken the lead in raising awareness on our campus. She called to tell me she had slashed her wrists and taken two bottles of pills.

She said to me on the phone, "I always thought when I reached the breaking point that it would be some big thing that pushed me over the edge. But it's not." Later at the hospital, while waiting for her father to arrive from out of town, she said to me, "What do I say when he asks me why I did it? 'Dad, I just don't fit in with the world?' "

As Jennifer convulsed in her hospital bed, her stomach torn to bits by the pills she had taken, I murmured, "I know, I know" and in fact I did know because—just like Jennifer—I took 140 aspirin one night in high school because I couldn't see a future for myself that offered any hope. I had never met an accomplished LGBT person, so I didn't have a model for a happy, successful life.

When you're an LGBTQ teenager, you don't need some big thing to push you over the edge, as Jennifer discovered. Every day of your life, you get the message that you just don't fit in. Sooner or later it hits home, as it did that afternoon with Jennifer, who everybody thought was so "together" with her student leadership position and her 1420 SAT score.

As we've seen, both LGBTQ young people who are out and those who are trying to hide their orientation face taunts, name calling, physical abuse and harassment every day of their lives. It gets so bad that, according to one study, as many as 28 percent of LGBTQ students drop out of high school because they just can't take it anymore. Those who stay in school need to figure out how to cope with their constant vulnerability, the undermining of their self-confidence, and the anticipation and fear of violence.

Unfortunately, many use unhealthy ways to escape. They self-medicate with drugs and alcohol, overeat or stop eating, fail to protect themselves from pregnancy and disease or turn inward and withdraw into depression. Many attempt suicide.

While these are very real and serious problems for LGBTQ teens, it is important not to pathologize all LGBTQ teens. Many adjust quite well and are "star students" and conversely, many overcompensate by being "star students" but may nevertheless be in pain. It is important that you understand that these problems are not an automatic result of being LGBTQ.

In this chapter I'll cover the serious risks that result when a child feels not only unsafe to express herself, but completely worthless and misunderstood. First, we'll discuss how to recognize the signs of depression, drug and alcohol abuse and eating disorders. Youth turn to drugs and alcohol to numb their pain and resort to eating disorders in an attempt to gain some control over their lives.

After we explore the "red flags" that indicate that a serious problem may be developing, I'll walk you through the process of communicating your concern to your child, finding appropriate help and preparing her for a consultation with a mental health professional, if needed.

Last, I'll alert you to the warning signs of suicide, a critical situation that requires immediate action. At the end of the chapter, we'll explore your feelings about this whole process to help you sort out your role and responsibilities.

With this information, you can be instrumental in getting your child the help she needs so she can grow up to be a happy, healthy, well-functioning adult.

SIGNS OF DEPRESSION

It's the drip, drip, drip of being out of step with the majority that wears LGBTQ youth down, as Jennifer told me from her hospital bed. No one even has to say anything bigoted. The ads, the commercials, the music all assume that everyone is straight. It's just the feeling that that there's something wrong with you and you're invisible and don't belong to the majority. (Remember the *Sesame Street* song, "One of these things is not like the others/One of these things doesn't belong?" That's what it feels like.)

It's exhausting, draining and depressing. And that's on top of the normal stresses of adolescence.

Keep in mind this destructive eroding of confidence and spirit as you read the traditional signs of depression that follow.

How to recognize the signs of depression

When teens become depressed, they don't act like depressed adults do. Depressed adults seem sad, move slowly, have little enthusiasm and a negative outlook on the world. They may complain, "I'm feeling blue" or "I'm so down."

Teens, on the other hand, may feel that way on the inside, but don't usually talk about it, especially to their parents. They show their unhappiness by changes in their mood and their behavior. If your child has two or more of the following eight signs for more than two consecutive weeks, there's a good chance she is depressed:

1. a change in school performance

2. inability to concentrate

3. irritability or anger

4. persistent unhappiness

5. change in eating or sleeping patterns

6. physical complaints

7. aggressive, impulsive or risk-taking behavior (drug or alcohol abuse)

8. talk of death or suicide.

While depressed adults often elicit sympathy from family members, having a depressed teen in the house often makes parents feel angry and frustrated. If you feel that way more than you usually do, that may be a sign as well.

It is important to recognize the signs of depression so it can be treated as soon as possible. The sooner treatment begins, the better the chances of recovery and the less likelihood that suicide will result. One in four youth who commit suicide do so during a period of major depression.[*]

SIGNS OF DRUG AND ALCOHOL ABUSE

Drug and alcohol abuse provide a fast and accessible escape for LGBTQ youth and helps them fit in, because it's a common "cool" interest. A study in Seattle public schools, for exam-

[*] Ryan and Futterman, p. 55.

ple, showed that 38.5 percent of LGBTQ youth admitted to heavy drug use, compared with 22.5 percent of their straight peers.

Brian's story is not uncommon. He recalls his high school days and his descent into the drug world: "Without the support of family, friends or teachers, and since my identity was invisible or only visible in negative ways, I soon turned to drugs and alcohol to escape my feelings of depression. What started as simple curiosity about what alcohol and cigarettes tasted and felt like, soon became a realization that such products could be used to make me happy, to hide my depression or to escape the depression that was plaguing my life.

> Legally available drugs include alcohol, prescribed medications, inhalants (fumes from glues, aerosols and solvents) and over-the-counter cough, cold, sleep and diet medications. The most commonly used illegal drugs are marijuana (pot), stimulants (cocaine, crack and speed), LSD, PCP, opiates, heroin and designer drugs (ecstasy).

"I soon surrounded myself with a new group of friends, many going through their own types of depression, who supported my habits and by the beginning of my senior year in high school I was having a shot of alcohol before school, and skipping out midday to drink up by the river. I soon started smoking pot, usually for the sole purpose to put me to sleep and avoid the hours of crying myself to sleep and contemplating suicide.

"Early in the school year, among one of my many 'drug' friends, I thought I'd found someone I could trust with my secret that I was gay. It didn't take long for this one person to tell most of his friends, who told their friends and so on.

"This new wave of problems and emotions led to even more severe depression with family and friends soon finding out, new harassment and torment, even death threats.

"Before long I turned to something stronger than alcohol and drugs to get my troubles out of my mind—if even temporarily.

My need for escape from my reality led down new roads lined with robo, poppers, acid, speed, ecstasy and cocaine. Each moving to the next as I found one stronger, better, lasting longer then the other—or I just needed something different."

Eventually, Brian learned that the solution to his problems could not be found in any drug. He explains where he did find the solution: "I found it in my family and friends, who wouldn't give up on me, though I already had. I found it in time and patience, both of which had been all but lost during my years using. And I found it in love and acceptance, from my friends and family, but more important, from me."

Like Brian, certain teenagers are at risk for developing serious alcohol and drug problems. They include the following four groups of teens:

1. those with a family history of substance abuse

2. those who are depressed

3. those who have low self-esteem

4. those who feel as if they don't fit in or are out of the mainstream.

Three out of four of these characteristics apply to many LGBTQ youth. If you sense that your child has these characteristics, then you should be particularly attuned to the following five warning signs of drug and alcohol abuse:

1. Physical: fatigue, repeated health complaints, red and glazed eyes and a lasting cough.

2. Emotional: personality change, sudden mood changes, irritability, irresponsible behavior, low self-esteem, poor judgment, depression and a general lack of interest.

3. Family: starting arguments, breaking rules or withdrawing from the family.

4. School: decreased interest, negative attitude, drop in grades, frequent absences, truancy and discipline problems.

5. Social problems: new friends who are less interested in standard home and school activities, problems with the law and changes to less conventional styles in dress and music.

Some of the warning signs listed above can also be signs of other problems. Don't necessarily jump to the conclusion that your child is abusing drugs. Once you recognize signs, proceed cautiously and follow the steps starting on page 269 for handling your concerns.

SIGNS OF EATING DISORDERS

One in ten teenage girls and young women suffer from eating disorders. As we discussed in Chapter 7, teenage girls who are questioning their sexuality often gain weight in an attempt to hide their developing breasts and hips.

Young women, who are questioning or lesbians, often have low self-esteem, which can make them vulnerable to developing an eating disorder. While obsessive, it does allow them to control one part of their life—their food intake—when so many aspects are beyond their control.

Is your child at risk?

According to Jean Bradley Rubel, Th.D., president of Anorexia Nervosa and Related Eating Disorders, Inc. (ANRED), the following four factors may contribute to eating disorders:

1. Biological Factors—People with obsessive compulsive personalities are more vulnerable to eating

disorders than others. New research suggests a biological base: that abnormal levels of brain chemicals predispose some people to anxiety, perfectionism and obsessive-compulsive thoughts and behaviors.

2. Psychological Factors—People with eating disorders tend to be perfectionists. They may have unrealistic expectations of themselves and others. In spite of their many achievements, they feel inadequate, defective and worthless. Eating disorders can be a female response to "the best little boy in the world" syndrome discussed earlier. They see everything as either good or bad, a success or a failure, fat or thin. If fat is bad and thin is good, then thinner is better and thinnest is best—even if thinnest is sixty-eight pounds in a hospital bed on life support.

3. Family Factors—Some people with eating disorders say they feel smothered in their families. Others feel abandoned, misunderstood and alone. Many lesbians feel this way, which makes them vulnerable to eating disorders. Parents who overvalue physical appearance can unwittingly contribute to an eating disorder; so can those who make critical comments, even in jest, about their children's bodies.

4. Social Factors—TV, movies and magazines flood teenagers with messages about the "advantages" of being thin. There is social pressure among teenage girls, in particular, to diet. Eating disorders often develop with dieting that gets carried to the extreme.

The two most common eating disorders are anorexia nervosa and bulimia. Following are warning signs you should be aware of for each.

Anorexia nervosa is an emotional disorder characterized by severe weight loss (or failure to gain weight). Teens with anorexia nervosa have an intense fear of becoming obese, even as they continue to lose weight. They severely restrict their calories, fast, exercise obsessively, use over-the-counter and prescription diet aids as well as diuretics and laxatives. They often "feel fat" even when they look emaciated.

The ten warning signs of anorexia nervosa include:

1. Significant and/or rapid loss of body weight

2. An obsession with dieting in spite of a thin frame

3. An intense fear of gaining weight

4. Amenorrhea (loss of menstrual cycle)

5. Unexplained hair loss

6. Cold or clammy hands and feet

7. Compulsive exercise habits, sometimes in a secretive fashion

8. Lying about food intake

9. Unexplained fainting

10. Periods of hyperactivity quickly followed by bouts of depression and anxiety

Bulimia is characterized by frequent episodes of binge eating followed by self-induced purging, often with the aid of laxatives, diuretics or vomiting-inducing drugs, to rid the body of food. Unlike anorectics, bulimics do not always appear thin.

The eight warning signs of bulimia include:

1. Eating large amounts of food uncontrollably

2. Abuse of laxatives or diuretics in a weight-loss effort

3. Shortness of breath, even after light activity

4. Making frequent trips to the bathroom after eating

5. A noticeable swelling and/or bloating, particularly in the glands of the neck and face

6. Visible tooth decay or dental problems, particularly in the front teeth

7. Bloodshot eyes or light bruising around upper cheek area

8. Irregular menstrual periods

WHEN TO BE CONCERNED

Once you have reviewed the list of warning signs for depression, drug and alcohol abuse and eating disorders, and determined which apply to your child, the following two clues will help you decide whether your concern is justified:

1. Try to gauge how long the warning signs have been going on.

2. Determine whether they interfere with your child's ability to function at home, school and with her friends.

Don't just look at grades, although plummeting grades are an indication of a problem. Look at other parts of her life as well. Did your son, a basketball fanatic for years, suddenly drop off the team without an explanation? Has your daughter pulled away from her clique of friends and now spends time in her room alone every day after school?

When you've observed these changes in behavior for at least two weeks, discuss your concerns with your spouse first, if you're married. See if he or she has noticed the same thing. If one of you feels it's a serious situation and the other says, "It's nothing. It'll pass," you may want to observe the situation for another week and then check in with each other again. If you're still at odds but one of you feels strongly that something is not right, go with that person's instinct, but sort out your differences in private before you approach your teen.

If you're a single parent, discuss your concerns with someone who knows your child well: her other parent, a grandparent, a neighbor or the parent of a friend of your child's. See if they have noticed similar changes or whether they have any worries. Your daughter may behave very differently when she's away from home. If they agree that her behavior is troubling, then discuss your concerns with your child.

COMMUNICATING YOUR CONCERN

Always obey the HALT rule—"Never speak when you're Hungry, Angry, Lonely or Tired"—for when (and when not) to raise sensitive issues. It's also not a good idea to initiate a conversation at the point of crisis. If your teen staggers in drunk at 1 a.m., that's not the time to have a serious discussion about the sudden change in her behavior. Wait until the next day, when you're not upset or pressed for time.

Approach her in a caring way, not with accusations and threats. You may be furious that she has been cutting school, but you don't want to begin with "What the hell's going on? Why aren't you going to school?" Instead, say, "I'd like to talk to you about something I'm concerned about," or "Do you have a few minutes? I have something on my mind." "Concern" is a good word to use because it conveys caring and is not judgmental.

Then talk about the behavior. You might say, "The school called again about your cutting out early. Let's talk about what's going on," or "You've come home drunk the last several Saturday nights. We need to talk about this." Don't ask her directly about whether she's depressed or whether something is wrong. Just express your concern, note the change in behavior and let her take it from there. If you need to ask a question, keep it open ended. Try not to ask a question that can be answered with "yes" or "no."

When she begins to talk, use the listening skills we discussed in Chapter 1. (Review them before your discussion if you need to.) She may be relieved that you've noticed something is wrong and blurt out, "I'm gay." She may tell you that she's being teased at school and can't take it anymore—that's why she cuts school. Or she may refuse to talk about what's going on now. In that case, encourage her to talk to another adult, such as a school counselor or favorite aunt, whom she feels comfortable with. Initially, you may feel rejected if this happens.

But remember that the most important thing is to find out what is causing the change in her behavior and if necessary, get her professional help.

Look at this discussion as the first of many. It may take more than one chat for her to open up. In the first discussion, she may tell you that she's being teased at school but not why. In a later talk, she may hint at the reason. It may take several more conversations for her to tell you why the kids are calling her names and how devastating it is for her.

Talking with your child can help prevent the kind of hopelessness and isolation that Tina, a seventeen-year-old lesbian, experienced: "A day in which the issue of sexual orientation is not mentioned or spoken about in school would be unusual. Every day I am forced to listen to the unaccepting or ignorant people around me. There seems to be no escape. Lately I've started to

lose hope altogether. It feels like nothing I can do will make a difference. If I confront the homophobia around me, it takes up all
my time and energy, and I feel totally alone in doing it. Furthermore, the students have no reason to listen to me. I am not a
teacher, not an adult. I don't have power here."

SEEKING HELP

The kind of help your teen needs depends on two factors:

1. the severity of the problem

2. the amount of support she has from family, friends
   and school officials.

Not every LGBTQ teenager needs professional help. In fact,
it's important not to suggest that first, particularly because society already has made your LGBTQ child feel that she's defective. If you suggest psychiatric or psychological intervention
quickly, you'll reinforce the notion that there is something wrong
with her. And now mom and dad think so, too.

The first step is to try to get your child peer support. Ask
her whether she knows if there is a gay-straight alliance at school
or a counselor she could talk to to find the names of other
LGBTQ students. Many teens are eager to connect with another
LGBTQ teen but may find it difficult to reach out themselves.
You can offer to make the phone calls for her if she's comfortable with that. Once she makes the connection with other
LGBTQ teens, monitor her behavior for a few weeks and see if
the situation gets any better. If it doesn't, then seek professional
help.

Some parents find that once their child comes out, the lies,
hiding and secrecy stop and so does the troubling behavior. For
others, like Tina, being out opens up the doors to a barrage of

further abuse. Tina may need more support than belonging to a gay-straight alliance at school, finding LGBT role models and reading LGBT authors. While all of these may help her feel less isolated and alone, she may still need counseling from a mental health professional.

Your child, too, may need a lot of support. The following three signs will tell you that she needs counseling:

1. If your child's behavior seems extreme to you and if you observe the warning signs often and consistently.

2. If you've tried to provide support and the pattern isn't changing or is getting worse. (She still sleeps thirteen hours a day or continues to cut school.)

3. If you have good communication between you, she may tell you verbally. She may say, "I can't take it any more" or "My life is unbearable."

FINDING THE RIGHT THERAPIST

There are two important steps in finding the right therapist for your child:

1. Getting a good referral

2. Checking out the therapist yourself.

You don't necessarily need to find an LGBT therapist but you do need to find someone who is comfortable with LGBTQ youth, who has had some experience working with them, and who is knowledgeable about the issues. I recommend that you check out several therapists ahead of time by yourself (without your child) so you can determine this. You don't want her to have a bad experience—given how loaded this issue is for so many.

And it may turn her off to the whole process of therapy as well as erode her trust in you, if you send her to someone with whom you haven't first connected.

The following five organizations are good places to get referrals:

1. Your local LGBT community centers referral service

2. A PFLAG meeting where other parents can recommend therapists who are good with LGBTQ youth

3. Your school guidance counselor, if he or she is receptive to such discussion

4. The National Association of Social Workers (NASW) for a list of their gay and lesbian caucuses. See Resources for the phone number.

5. The American Psychological Association in Washington, D.C., for a local referral. See Resources for phone number.

Once you have several names, make appointments to see them so you can check them out. When you meet with the therapist, explain why you feel your child needs to see someone. You can say something like, "I'm concerned about Jimmy. He has come home drunk the last few weekends and he's just come out at school. I think he needs help in sorting out his feelings." Tell her also that you are meeting with several therapists to find a good "fit" for your child—that is, someone who is experienced in gender and orientation issues and sensitive to the concerns of LGBTQ teens. Try to get a sense of whether she takes your concerns seriously. If she make comments like, "Well, all kids get teased" or "Your child is just going through a phase. I wouldn't worry about it," that is a sign that she would not be the right therapist, because she would belittle your child's concerns.

Then use the following questions as a guide to determine how comfortable and experienced she is with youth that have sexual orientation issues. Of course, add your own questions as well.

- What is your past experience with people who are LGBTQ? With LGBTQ youth in particular?
- What do you believe causes homosexuality? If she talks about a neurotic family background causing it, she is not well informed with the latest facts.
- Do you believe therapy can change someone's orientation? If she does, you want to find another therapist. That is not the purpose of your child's seeing her and should not be your hidden agenda either.
- What do you see as the cause of problems of LGBTQ youth: rejection and victimization or their homosexual orientation? If she feels your child's problem is due to her orientation, she will try to change it.
- What kind of professional training have you had to work with adolescents, LGBTQ people, or both?

There are also more subtle signs that a mental health professional has an accepting attitude to LGBTQ students. They include the following three tip-offs:

1. LGBT-positive posters, announcements of LGBT-related events or "Safe Zone" stickers in her office

2. The use of inclusive language and references to LGBTQ people in conversation

3. The use of nongendered pronouns when referring to student relationships, such as not calling a boy's girlfriend "she" and using the word "partner."

If you feel satisfied with the therapist's answers and by what you observe in her language and demeanor, tell her you want to discuss your consultation with your child and will get back to her.

Go through this same process with two or three other therapists. Choose therapists of both genders, so you can give your child a choice. Some youth only want to see someone of the same gender; others are struggling so much with their attraction to the same gender that the last thing they want to do is see someone of their gender. By the time you talk with your child about the need to see a mental health professional, you should have two or three names of therapists whom you feel good about.

PREPARING YOUR CHILD FOR A MENTAL HEALTH CONSULTATION

Plan ahead how and when you will broach the subject of seeing a mental health professional with her. I can't repeat often enough how crucial it is to carefully pick a quiet time to talk when you are both fairly calm, as I've stressed for every important discussion.

Lead into the discussion with a general comment, such as, "I'd like to talk to you about something" or "There's something on my mind. Have a few minutes?" Then, bring up your concern. You can say something like, "A few weeks ago, we talked about your drinking/cutting school. I know you tried to connect with other gay kids at school but I'm still concerned about your drinking (or that you're still cutting school). I know you're dealing with a lot—you've just come out, your friends are adjusting to this, people are not welcoming at school. It's a lot for anybody. You've tried to get support at school, but it doesn't seem to be enough. I think you'd find it easier to manage if you got more support. I'd like you to see a therapist."

You can add, "I want you to be a happy, healthy person and I know somebody who can help you learn how to cope with some of the understandable difficulties you're encountering in your life right now. That's what I'm trying to do for you."

If you've been in therapy yourself, you might also share a personal experience. Talk about the times you needed extra support and how therapy helped you. Learning that others they respect have worked with therapists and found them helpful can be a tremendous relief to teens who think only "crazy" people go to a therapist.

Unfortunately, many youth attach stigma to therapy. If she worries that kids at school will find out, explain that the sessions are confidential and no one will know unless she chooses to tell them.

If your child retorts, "I'm not crazy. I don't need a shrink," ask her what she has heard about mental health professionals and try to dispel myths with facts.

Make four things very clear:

1. You are not trying to "fix" her and the therapist is not going to try to change her orientation or make her straight.

2. There is nothing wrong with her and she is not crazy.

3. She is not bad or weak. It's the strong, healthy person who asks for help when she needs it. This is a particularly important message to give to boys because they tend to see people who go to psychiatrists as wimps.

4. The purpose is to get extra support and to give her more coping skills.

If she balks and says, "I'm fine. I can cope alone. I don't need to talk to anyone," then repeat again, "Well, I'm very concerned about you and . . . (again insert the problem behavior: your drinking, your cutting school, etc.) and would like you to see someone."

Then say, "Let me just tell you about the therapists I've checked out for you. I'd like you to agree to meet with them once and see how it goes." Of course, you cannot force a teenager to see someone. You need her consent and cooperation, but getting her in the door and connecting with a therapist is the first step.

Then one by one, go through the names of the therapists you've checked out and tell her why you think each would be a good match for her. Stay with the discussion until she agrees to see one for a consultation. If she still insists that she doesn't want to see someone, ask her to think about it overnight and you'll talk again tomorrow.

If you feel therapy is essential and your child remains resistant, sometimes it may be necessary to give you child a hard choice, along the lines of "If you can't agree to seek help, I'll have to take steps to make sure you're safe, such as taking away your driving privileges or instituting an earlier curfew so you aren't out drinking and driving."

Make it clear that the child has a choice here, and that the consequence of that choice are her responsibility, and hers alone. Once in therapy, many youth find it valuable. Getting them to take that first step, though, can be a struggle.

SUICIDE

According to the Centers for Disease Control/Massachusetts Department of Education Youth Risk Behavior Survey, done in 1999, 33 percent of LGBTQ youth will attempt suicide during their adolescence—well over four times the rate of their heterosexual peers.

That means your child is in a high risk group for suicide.

Jared's story will illustrate how very common suicidal thoughts are among LGBTQ teens. Now twenty, Jared thought about suicide at many points in high school. He remembers, "There was a time in my life where a day wouldn't go by that I didn't want to kill myself because I just felt so isolated and so alone. Every problem seemed ten times bigger at that time. The smallest thing would happen and it was like, oh the world's going to end. I was severely depressed in tenth grade."

He explains what his depression was about: "I was trying to figure out how I fit into the world and I just felt like I didn't fit. I mean I knew there were other gay people out there, but I didn't know who they were. I didn't see any and I didn't know any, so of course, I felt alone."

Jared continues, "Every day, I thought, how am I going to do it? I can remember at one point going to the library and writing a will, deciding who I wanted to give my stuff to and who I'd say my last good-byes to. I never came to actually doing it but I just felt that bad. I just wanted everything to end. I couldn't take it anymore.

"At the time I had to come to terms with I'm not getting married. I guess I'm not going to have kids. I guess I'm not going to do anything. My whole world was shattered because growing up this is what they teach you—that you're going to grow up and get a job and you're going to get married, have kids and raise a family. Now granted, people don't necessarily have to do that but that is so ingrained in you that to wake up and realize, oh, my God, I can't do this. So what do I do? You just don't know."

Jared lived with his depression and suicidal thoughts for almost a year. The turning point came when he confided in a guidance counselor that he wanted to die. With his counselor's support, he started telling people he was gay. Unburdened of his secret and supported by his friends, his depression began lifting. Life didn't seem so bleak.

Unique Stressors

Studies show that between 48 and 76 percent of LGBTQ youth are like Jared—despondent and depressed and contemplating suicide but they don't actually attempt it. Between 29 and 42 percent of LGBTQ youth, however, do attempt suicide (The rate for adolescents in general ranges from 6 to 13 percent).*

In this section, I'm going to point out the particular stressors on LGBTQ youth, alert you to the warning signs of suicide and tell you what to do in case of emergency.

Some of the risk factors for LGBTQ youth are similar to those for all adolescents. They include:

- low self-esteem
- family conflict
- substance abuse
- a past suicide attempt
- a history of attempted or completed suicides among friends or family members.

In addition, there are three stressors unique to LGBTQ youth that make them particularly vulnerable. They are†:

1. Their increasing awareness of same-sex attractions. Most suicide attempts are made between the time a teen is aware of her same-gender feelings and the time she discloses them to others or establishes a positive LGBT identity. That is a period of extreme loneliness, isolation and self-doubt.
2. The disclosure of their sexual orientation to family and friends. Those who attempt suicide are less likely to

---

* Russell, Stephen I. and Kara Joyner, Ph.D., p. 1276.
† Hershberger, Scott, Neil W. Pilkingon, and Anthony R. D'Augelli, p. 479.

have supportive parents and a support system of friends. Again, isolation and rejection play a part in motivating suicide attempts.

3. Victimization provoked by their sexual orientation. Constantly living with verbal abuse, threats of physical abuse, and violence erode teens' self-esteem, increase their sense of isolation and can lead to increased depression. The more teens depart from the typical male and female behavior and dress, the more their peers will reject them and the more isolated they will feel. This is particularly a problem for trans teens.

Warning Signs

If your child has some of the risk factors listed above, including those for all youth and those particular to LGBTQ youth, she is vulnerable to suicide. In addition, three warning signs indicate that your child has serious intentions of attempting suicide. These put your child at immediate risk and must be dealt with at once. They are[*]:

1. If your child seems preoccupied with death or suicide in the following three areas:
   • poetry, essays or other writing
   • the music she listens to or plays
   • her conversations
   Any talk of suicide must be taken seriously. These are not idle threats or scare tactics. Typical comments include "I wish I were dead," "You won't have to worry about me anymore" or "Soon I'll be out of your hair for good." Don't dismiss these as idle talk. Address them directly to see if they represent something deeper.

2. If your child starts giving away prized possessions. If she

[*] Shapiro, Patricia G., pp. 125–126.

hands out her favorite CDs, posters of rock stars, or special mementos, that is a serious signal that she is thinking of ending her life.

3. If your child has a plan. If she has thought about the following, that constitutes an emergency and requires immediate intervention:
   - when she will end her life
   - how she will carry out her plan
   - where the suicide will take place

What to Do in an Emergency

If your child shows any of the above three warning signs, you must question her directly about whether she's thinking of suicide. Child psychiatrist Lawrence L. Kerns, M.D., states clearly in his book, *Helping Your Depressed Child*, "Talking about suicide will not plant an idea in a child who isn't suicidal and it won't cause suicide in one who is."

Not recognizing that your child is in distress can have serious consequences.

If your child shows you several poems she has written that are very dark and concerned with dying, if she makes some of the comments suggested above or if she starts giving her friends her sports trophies, express your concern and note the behavior. Say, "I'm concerned about you. You seem so preoccupied with death and dying lately" or "I'm worried about you. You're giving away all your favorite things." Then let her respond, keeping in mind that her actions may be cries for help.

Then you must take the conversation one step further. Take a deep breath and ask, "Are you thinking of hurting yourself?" or "Do you ever think of killing yourself?"

If she says, "I am down lately but I'd never hurt myself," you can feel more at ease that she won't do something now. But she must still be evaluated by a mental health professional as soon as possible. You do not have time to follow the guidelines I outlined earlier in the chapter for how to select a mental health professional. This situation requires immediate action, so call one of the following at once:

- your family physician for a referral
- a crisis hotline
- a suicide prevention center

Follow the same procedure if your child admits she is contemplating suicide.

Ask your teen to establish a contract with you that she won't hurt herself until she talks to you or to a counselor. Be very firm about this. If she says, "I'll try" or "maybe" that means she is still in danger.

If she won't make a contract with you, ask her if she has a plan. Notice how detailed the plan is. If she has thought through how she'll do it, what method she'll use and where she'll do it, contact a mental health professional immediately.

While you are waiting for help, do the following*:

- Encourage her to talk. Ask her, "Tell me what you're thinking about or what scares you or what bothers you." Use every listening skill we've discussed in this book. In addition, follow these three "don'ts":

1. **Don't** judge her.

2. **Don't** deny her reality by saying, "Oh, it's not really that bad." This is how she feels now. If she says, "Things are so bad at school, I just don't want to live," say something like, "I know you're feeling low now and it feels like things won't get better, but they will. We need to ride out this rough time."

---

* Shapiro, Patricia G., pp. 127–128.

3. **Don't** tell her how much she has to look forward to or how much fun she'll have next summer on her trip. Stay with her feelings.

• Tell your child how much you love her and how much you'd miss her if she were gone. Say this repeatedly. Trapped in their own pain, many adolescents don't realize that suicide is forever and aren't thinking about the impact of their decision on others. You can say, "Ending your life will stop your pain, but my pain and that of your dad and sister will continue. With you gone, there's nothing we can do to end our pain. We love you. You are an important part of our family." This kind of conversation can be a wake-up call to teens who think no one cares.

And if you are a parent who thinks that talk of suicide or even an attempt is just a way to get attention, that should be a wake-up call to *you* to do just that: give her the attention and TLC she craves.

• State your personal stand on suicide. Tell her that "Suicide is not an acceptable option." Remind her that there are many other ways to manage problems and feelings and that together you'll figure out those when she's feeling better.

• If your child refuses to talk with you, tell her you want her to talk to someone and ask her whom she'd like you to call. It could be a grandparent, another relative, a teacher or counselor. Try not to take this as a personal rebuff. The most important thing is that she talks to someone she trusts.

• Do not leave her alone. You or another family member must stay with her until she is in a safe setting.

• Take all guns and medication out of the house. This includes over-the-counter medications, such as aspirin, sleeping pills and cold medications, which can be deadly taken in large doses.

If Your Child Has Attempted Suicide

If your child has made a suicide attempt, take her to the closest emergency room immediately. Make sure that she talks to a mental health professional in addition to getting medical care. At some point, you, too, should be part of the discussion so that everyone in the family can understand why this has happened and can prevent it from happening again.

Because a suicide attempt is so frightening to both parents and teens, there is a tendency to deny the seriousness of what happened. Your child may say, "I'm fine now. I won't do it again."

And parents, wanting to believe that the situation is not so serious, may agree and say, "She didn't really mean to hurt herself."

This is just not so. A suicide attempt reflects unresolved problems that still exist after the attempt. If the issues are not dealt with, they will remain and can resurface, possibly in another attempt. Before you leave the hospital, make sure your child has a referral for a mental health professional.

MOVING FORWARD

That your child has serious problems is no doubt very distressing to you. Of course, you're concerned about her well-being but you may also feel guilty, responsible, confused and frightened. You may feel that you have failed as a parent. These are all natural responses that many parents experience in similar circumstances.

The important thing now is to keep your child healthy and to give her the support she needs to stay strong mentally, physically and emotionally. Here's how:

- Find a good support system for yourself. Talk to your spouse, a close friend or a PFLAG parent about your feelings, concerns and fears that arose from the suicide attempt. Don't put these on your child.
- Help your child find a support system.

Encourage her to find LGBT friends, join a gay-straight alliance or find another LGBT-friendly group in the community.

- Encourage her to stay in counseling until she feels she has worked out her issues.
- Don't micromanage your child's life, but continue to tune in to her behavior, so you can recognize the signs and symptoms of serious problems should they resurface.
- Recognize that recovery takes time. Be patient with your child, and yourself.

Chapter Eleven

YOUNG PEOPLE
SPEAK TO PARENTS

THROUGHOUT THIS BOOK, I've tried to give you a sense of what it's like to be an LGBTQ teen in today's world. You've heard their conflicts and struggles, their fears and their anxieties. But nowhere in the book have youth talked directly to you, their parents. That is the goal of this chapter: for your sons and daughters to tell you in their own voices and with their own words the following:

1. What teens wish their parents knew about their lives

2. Questions teens wish their parents would ask

3. Teenagers' advice for parents

The teens whose voices you'll hear in this chapter come from all across the country, from small towns and large cities, from welcoming environments and hostile ones. I have not given identifying information about the speakers of the quotes because the details don't really matter here. The comments could come from anyone, and in many cases, similar comments were repeated again and again, regardless of race, class, gender or age.

In every instance, I've used the teenagers' quotes verbatim and only made changes to correct spelling or grammatical errors.

When you finish reading this chapter, you will know what your LGBTQ child needs and wants to feel sincerely supported.

I. WHAT TEENS WISH THEIR PARENTS KNEW ABOUT THEIR LIVES

Some of the teens' wishes are so simple that you may wonder how anyone could have missed something so obvious, yet it is often difficult to see clearly someone we are so close to or have known for so long. Many speak to their deep need to be loved and accepted for who they are—not an easy thing for many parents to do.

What do you wish your parents knew about your life?
 • "I wish my mother and my father could see how people treat me—people that I don't even know. I wish they could experience the grief and sorrow, the fear, that I feel every day. I wish they knew how hard I try every day to get just one person to stop using 'gay' as a derogatory remark. I wish they knew how suicidal I once was, how much I used to cut myself, and how hard I try NOT to cut myself when I get terribly mad or upset."
 • "In coming out to my parents over the past year, I had almost wished that they had stopped talking to me, because it is much harder to be hated by the people you love, especially when they are right in your face."
 • "My family has a history of being 'military men.' Since I am the only male in my family, Dad expects me to follow in his footsteps. Every day I hear 'Be a real man. Be a marine.' I wish my parents would create an environment where I could be honest with them and tell them I'm gay."
 • "I really want my parents to know that I am gay. Three

weeks before the date I had picked to come out, my cousin re-vealed that he is gay. My grandmother took to her bed for three weeks and my dad put his arm around me and said how grateful he was that he had a 'normal son.' Needless to say, I haven't told them I'm gay. If I had one wish, I'd wish that my parents would realize that regardless of my sexual orientation, I am the son that they love and trust."

• "I wish they knew that I'm still Tim even though I'm gay. I wish they knew that I'm not going to die at thirty due to AIDS or hepatitis, merely because I am gay. I wish they knew that I'm in love with a wonderful boy named Jim, and that being gay isn't going to make me a societal outcast or a failure or even a hair-dresser. I wish they would at least try to understand me."

• "I wish my parents could truly understand how happy I am. I wish I didn't feel weird about telling them things about myself and my boyfriend and that I didn't feel like I shouldn't show af-fection in front of them."

• "These are things which I had to make clear to my parents after they read my journal and found out that I am gay:

1. Your child is not a pedophile.

2. Your child is not the victim of a pedophile.

3. Your child will not get beaten up.

4. Your child is not sleeping with every other gay teenager within a fifty-mile radius.

5. Your child (as long as you have reared him prop-erly) is not infected with AIDS.

6. Your child is not a pariah.

7. Ask your child what he wants you to do. Unwanted advice/'assistance' can turn out to be a hindrance and a major pain in the ass.

8. It's not your fault.

9. It's not your child's fault.

10. Just chill; your child is no different from the day before he came out to you."

. • "Every teen, gay or not, does not want their parents to know much about their lives. To claim our independence from them, I think teens try to maintain as much separation from our parents as possible. Gay teens in particular . . . almost have to keep more things secret from their parents—to either ensure their safety or to be fully sure of their sexuality before they come out to their parents."

• "I wish my parents knew that they say more hurtful things to me and are meaner in one fight than I get from anyone and everyone in all my school years combined."

• "It would be great if my mother would let me go [to gay support groups], and furthermore take me to gay support groups in the area as eagerly as she takes me to lacrosse practice."

• "I wish I could be open with them about my bisexuality, but they have always been so judgmental. I have hinted to my mother about my orientation, but she says, 'D . . . , you know how I feel about that!' or 'You better not be!' "

• "I am a depressed, anxious, attention-deficit-disorder kind of girl—with a pretty smile to cover it up. All it would take for me to share it with her is her to ask. To talk to me about something other than what I did today, what I'm doing tomorrow and whether I'm cleaning my room."

• "I only wish my parents could see my happiness and would want to be a part of that, instead of being ashamed of the one they once took so much pride in. I want them to meet my girl, get to know her for the person she is, instead of what takes place behind CLOSED bedroom doors. I just want to feel loved again . . . if only for a short while."

II. QUESTIONS TEENS WISH THEIR PARENTS WOULD ASK

Parents are always asking their kids questions, but they're generally not the questions teens *wish* their parents would ask. The following section will give you clues to the kinds of questions that would help teens open up and share more of their lives with you.

What questions do you wish your parents would ask you?

• "I wish my parents, especially my mom, would ask me the one question that I dread and yet desire: 'Are you gay?' She thinks I have an open relationship with her, that I tell her almost everything. I tell her everything but the most important part of me—I'm a lesbian, I'm attracted to girls."

• "I would have loved for them to ask me if I was dating someone, because all through high school I couldn't talk to my parents about people I was dating, and I thought they thought I couldn't get a date. That really hurt my self-esteem."

• "None really, I would just like them to know that I am living a very troublesome life right now, and as happy as I may seem, I hide my emotions because I get shut out if I try to share my feelings."

• "They could have asked me *some* questions about my life. Instead, every conversation we had, was about *them*. They seemed never to be interested in me. I played softball for six years and they never appeared at one game."

• "I wish they asked me questions to dispel the myths their generation taught them before they throw those kinds of lies in my face in the heat of the moment."

• "Are you okay? Are you happy? Are you sad? Can we come to see your play? Can we do anything to help out? Are you gay? (As opposed to 'I looked in your journal, I know you're gay.') Basically, anything beyond 'Are you hungry?' "

• "I want my parents to ask me, 'Are you gay?' And I want to shout, 'No, but I'm bisexual!' "

III. TEENAGERS' ADVICE FOR PARENTS

How often have you felt like telling your teenager, "Just tell me what to do and I'll do it"? Of course, these issues cannot be remedied with a quick solution. Nonetheless, here you'll hear directly from teens about just what they would like from you, their parents.

What advice do you have for your parents?

• "Create an environment for kids to explore their sexuality, BUT, do not be overly pushy with that. My mother asked me if I was gay way before I was ready to talk about it. And she didn't ask in a way that was supportive. It was more hostile than that."

• "Everyone loves their parents. If you let us warm up to you, it will be easier for us to talk and share. Although this may be hard to accept, we may not share every detail with you—trust me, this is for the better!"

• "Take time to remember how you felt as a teenager with your parents."

• "It would have been wonderful if my parents had read literature about having a gay child, because their not doing so made it seem as though they didn't take me seriously when I came out to them. It made me feel as though they thought it was a phase."

• "I would like my parents to stop thinking this is all going to change, and that I am being so loud. They think I am too vocal, too proud. 'Oh, being gay isn't who you are, it's a part of you.' If my mother thought about it, how big is being heterosexual a part of her life? It's big. And my pride is what has kept my head out of the noose. I wish they would just accept the fact that I will never be straight."

- "I want them to attend PFLAG meetings and learn more about me."
- "Please try and look past the outer shell of your child—past the gay, past the stigma of being gay. Look at your baby, the one you have raised and love so much. Being gay is nothing more than a feeling. It does not change who they are. It may change the way they act but not their hearts. Also please ask questions, I am glad my mom did. She has become a pillar of support in my life."
- "Understand that this is real love, not lust."
- "Just stop thinking it's going to change. Stop telling me to ignore it or be tough. Because It doesn't work when you forever are hearing 'fag' and 'faggot' in the hallways and in class."
- "I accept my sexual orientation, but would like to feel secure enough to tell my parents I'm a lesbian. In order for that to happen, we'll have to find an opportunity to sit down together for more than fifteen minutes. I love my parents very much, but it seems to me they are too busy with their social lives to notice that I really need them."
- "Be selfless. Coming out is hard and although no one wants their son/daughter to be gay, no one even wants to be gay let alone have parents not accept them. It is a difficult process for both parent and child. The more supportive the parent is, the easier it is for the child."
- "Clothes do not determine sexual orientation or gender."
- "Just because you don't want your son/daughter to go to a pride festival, support group or gay friend's house, it doesn't mean you shouldn't let them go. The more you tell your son/daughter they can't go here, wear this or do that, the more they're going to want to or sneak around you to do so."
- "I wish we had spent more time doing quality activities together when I was young and they accepted me for who I was instead of always encouraging me to be exactly like them when they were my age."

• "While other kids were annoyed by their curfews and over-protective parents, I never had any of that. My parents didn't care what I did. We never had 'the drug talk' or 'the sex talk.' I think the most important thing parents can do for their kid, LGBT or not, is take an active interest in their life but not force themselves into it where they are not wanted."

• "I wish my mom could understand that I'm not trans to hurt her, that by rejecting my female body I'm not rejecting her but rather just finally admitting I have body parts that aren't right for me."

• "I understand that getting used to these issues will take my mom a while, but I wish she could understand how hard it is for me to be her therapist. It's one thing to want to be honest with me day-to-day, that's cool. But truly, if she's not going to respond positively to me and my identity, I wish she could take that somewhere else."

• "Please, when we tell you we are gay, don't stand up and shout, 'WHAT?!' It only makes some of us more reluctant to tell you anything in the future."

WHAT TEENS FEAR HEARING MOST

Certain comments and questions will drive your child away and push him further into the closet. They include the following, culled from actual comments that parents made to LGBTQ children:

> "Are you still gay?"
> "I'm sure it's just a phase that you'll outgrow."
> "You're just a follower."
> "If your father were alive, he'd die again."
> "Are you sure you don't want to see a doctor?"
> "How do you know for sure?"
> "Thank God your brother isn't gay too. If he were, I'd kill myself."

• "My mother tries to please everyone in our family and making an image of perfection for everyone outside of it. It's funny—she's stuck with a daughter who's queer. She loves me. I just can't relate to her. She nags me about everything. Maybe I'll send her a card . . . 'Mom, please stop being fake. I love you and I would like to get to know what the *real* you is like. Happy Mother's Day.'"

• "I just want to be loved. Is that so wrong?"

Chapter   Twelve

CONCLUSION

Throughout this book, I've written a lot about my experiences growing up LGBTQ and the kinds of difficulties and challenges I've experienced. But I haven't written much about my relationship with my own mother and how she came to accept me as a gay man.

That story is a fitting conclusion for this book, because if my mother, who grew up in the rural South during the Depression without much formal education, came to accept me, you can do the same with your child.

I hope this story, which began when I was a young boy and culminated in 2000 when I was thirty-seven years old, will give you hope and inspiration.

My father, a Southern Baptist minister, died when I was eight, so I grew up alone with my mom because my four siblings, who are much older, had all moved out of the house by the time I was in sixth grade. I already knew at that point that I was gay, but no one else did.

Having pretty much only my mom, one of the most important things for me as a child was to please her. I knew education was very important to her, so I worked hard and stayed in school even though it was a horrible place for me.

I graduated from high school in 1981. I couldn't wait to get out of town and to begin my life. In college, I would be free of my hometown, free of my school and free of my mom. I'd be able to have a life. I went to college up north and came out to her for good in 1982 at the beginning of my sophomore year in college.

But from that time on, we had a strained relationship.

To avoid the potential of being hurt, I distanced myself from her. I didn't come home often. I didn't talk to her much because she was having trouble dealing with me. And I didn't want to feel her disappointment. We talked about the weather a lot, because she didn't want to hear about my life. Before I came out, she wanted to meet my friends, but no longer.

To her credit, she realized in the late 1980s that she was losing her son and started seeing a therapist. The therapist suggested she find some other parents to talk to in the same situation. She did—by founding a PFLAG chapter in Winston-Salem, my hometown, in 1988. She started the chapter with the help of a therapist who referred people she counseled to my mother.

But that's not the end of the story.

In October 2000, the public school system in Winston-Salem held a mandatory training for all guidance counselors on LGBT issues. It came about through the insistence of our local GLSEN chapter, which lobbied for it for a year. I was invited to come home to do that training. Simultaneously, the local Unitarian church, which is a mile from the Baptist church I grew up in, invited me to be the guest minister the day before this training.

In my sermon, which I called "Faith of My Father and Mother," I contrasted the darkness and fear associated with the faith of my father, the Southern Baptist religion, with the hope and empowerment I received at the altar of my mother's faith, education.

A couple of weeks before I went home I had said to my therapist, "You know, pretty much everything is resolved in my life. I'm getting to go home. I've made the world a better place in my hometown. I've been accepted by my mom and I've worked out all the demons from my childhood."

He asked, "Is there anything you would want that you don't have?"

I said, "I just wish that someone would say they are sorry for what I went through."

So, back to North Carolina, I did that sermon Sunday morning and the training the next day. On Tuesday morning I had a 7:00 a.m. flight back to New York. I'm sitting at the dining room table having a quick coffee with my mom at 5 a.m. I get up to leave and my mom says, "Sit down. I have something to say to you."

Annoyed, I said, "What's that? I've gotta go."

My mom said, "I just wanted to tell you two things. First of all, I am so sorry I wasn't there for you when you were a kid and you were going through all of this awful stuff in school. I'm really sorry I wasn't there for you."

She continued, "The second thing I want you to know is that I'm so proud of you for doing what you're doing, so kids today don't have to go through what you went though."

First of all, I thought these kinds of scenes only happen in movies—people just don't get to hear the words they've waited their whole lifetime to hear, except in Hollywood's fantasies. Then I thought of all the years that my mother and I had lost because of homophobia, years in which we distanced ourselves from each other because we didn't know how to talk about my being gay in the right way. I thought of my incredible luck to have a mother who, without the benefit of a book like this or much in the way of resources, finally did make that journey and did come out of this tunnel on the right side.

I realized then that I have something that a lot of LGBT people don't have: I know that I am fully loved and fully embraced by my mother for who I am and what I do.

All of us, whether we're LGBTQ or straight, whether we're seventeen or thirty-seven or fifty-seven, profoundly crave that level of approval and acceptance from our parents. I so wish that my story would become a typical one that all LGBTQ children—in fact, all children—experience. And not when they're thirty-seven but when they're teenagers.

I hope that this book will shorten the lag time for you and your child.

On those days when my faith in the capacity of people to learn and grow wavers, I look to my mom. Raised in segregation, she has embraced her African American daughter-in-law. Raised with homophobia, she founded the first PFLAG chapter in North Carolina, and regularly attends the meetings of one of the newest GLSEN chapters, GLSEN/Winston-Salem. Raised to turn her back on those deemed "unclean," she spends three days a week volunteering at Holly Haven, the first hospice for people with AIDS in Winston-Salem, a facility in which each resident is Black.

When I am feeling overwhelmed with the struggles young people face every day, I picture my seventy-five-year-old mother holding the hands of a seventy-pound African American man with AIDS as he passes from this life to the next. And I am restored.

If my mom could do it, you can do it.

Here's the irony, though: Even though homophobia cost us many years of estrangement, in the end it became the basis of my having a much stronger relationship with my mother than most of my siblings do. She and I have had to be more real and more authentic with each other and face more issues honestly than my other siblings have with our mom.

In the end, because my mother was willing to grow, homophobia ended up being a blessing that made our relationship better.

Ultimately, all parents want that sense of real connection with their child. Believe it or not, your child coming out might even give you the chance to have it more than if he had not been LGBTQ. Your child's coming out is an opportunity, not a burden or a curse. Your child is giving you a chance to know who he really is and to forge a real connection with him based on authenticity.

You have a rare opportunity within your grasp.

GUIDELINES FOR TAKING LEGAL ACTION

In Chapter 9, I discussed how to advocate for your child at school. In my experience, litigation should be the last resort, not the first. If you decide to take legal action, review the following suggestions.

WHEN TO SUE

I recommend you sue only under the following two circumstances:

1. If you've exhausted all ways of negotiation and they're not working

2. If your child is in immediate physical and/or emotional danger

In both cases, the school system has been unsupportive and litigation seems to be the only way to compel it to take action. In our litigious society we often use suing to resolve every single issue. I'd urge you to try to work with the system to institute the kinds of changes needed, and look to litigation only if that fails.

Once the issue has moved out of the hands of the educators and into the hands of the lawyers and the politicians, you're moving away from people who theoretically have your child's best interest at heart. On the legal stage, the needs of youth and parents take a back seat to the legal proceedings. Parents who have taken the litigation route tell me they feel as if they have turned over their child and his well-being to some system that they have no control over, no knowledge of and no understanding of.

This, combined with the sometimes-lengthy time frame of litigation, can be very discouraging. Lawsuits are at times appropriate, but it has been my experience that those times are rare, and that the threat of one is often as effective for making change happen as actually filing one.

COURT RULINGS

As of this writing, only four states—Massachusetts, Connecticut, Wisconsin and California—have education codes that protect young people from harassment in sexual orientation. Minnesota and New Jersey have broad antidiscrimination laws where students are similarly protected, as schools are designated "public accommodations" which the law covers. Vermont and Washington state have antiharassment laws that protects students from harassment based on sexual orientation. But the laws are constantly changing. By the time you read this, hopefully more states will have laws in effect.

Massachusetts set the stage when Republican Governor William Weld and his Governor's Commission on Gay and Lesbian Youth and Massachusetts activists created a foundation for the "Safe Schools" movement in 1993. They added "sexual orientation" to the state's education code, fought for teacher training, lobbied the State Board of Education to recommend that each high school have a gay-straight alliance, and then secured state funds to support them, thus establishing the first statewide program to combat anti-LGBT bias in schools. Massachusetts has been an inspiration for activists around the nation who have initiated similar efforts based on its model.

For the most up-to-date information on current laws and legislation, consult the following web sites:

- Lambda Legal Defense and Education Fund: www.lambdalegal.org
- American Civil Liberties Union: www.aclu.org
- The National Center for Lesbian Rights: www.nclrights.org
- Gay and Lesbian Advocates and Defenders: www.glad.org

IF YOU DECIDE TO SUE

Before you enter the litigation process, keep in mind three things:

1. PREPARE FOR A LONG HAUL. Litigation often takes years to make its way through the courts. Former Boy Scout James Dale spent a decade in the courts seeking redress after getting dismissed because he was gay (and still lost). Lawsuits often are extended efforts, and it is important that you brace yourself for that long and winding road (and the unexpected dips and turns it takes) before heading down it.

2. KNOW WHAT YOUR GOAL IS. Before you begin, decide what you hope to achieve with your lawsuit by exploring with an attorney the strengths and weaknesses of the case and what is realistic. What you ask for should correspond to the strength of your case.

    For some, simply fighting back is gratification enough, and the eventual decision of the court (yea or nay) is secondary to reclaiming one's voice. Others have very specific demands, such as nonmonetary justice, like a formal apology or better policies with meaningful trainings to implement them. There may be points in the litigation where the other side makes you a counter-offer and you may have to make a decision.

In order to do so effectively, I urge you to go in knowing the following three things:

1. what you hope to win (your best case scenario)

2. what you'd settle for

3. what is unacceptable to you.

This information will help you navigate the various decision points you may face as the process unfolds.

3. UNDERSTAND THAT YOU ARE IN A DIFFERENT WORLD NOW. Courts do not make laws: They interpret and enforce them. This may mean that what seems "right" to a member of the general public is not "right" in a courtroom. In the absence of an inclusive non-discrimination law or other legal basis for action, a judge who personally thinks what has happened to your child is wrong may still be forced to rule against you. Similarly, some judges may be totally unconvinced by a legal argument that seems airtight to you and your family. This can be incredibly frustrating and hard to understand or accept.

But the fact is: When we enter litigation, legal principles now govern the course of events. That is a critical but difficult leap to make for those of us who are not lawyers.

The law can be a powerful ally for parents seeking to compel schools to "do the right thing" for their children. But litigation can also be a double-edged sword, and parents are advised to wield it carefully. Take the above factors into careful consideration as you make your decision on whether to take legal action on your child's behalf.

BIBLIOGRAPHY

Beal, Anne and Robert J. Sternberg., editors. *The Psychology of Gender.* New York and London: Guilford Press, 1993.

Bernstein, Robert A. *Straight Parents, Gay Children: Keeping Families Together.* New York: Thunder's Mouth Press, 1995.

Bono, Chastity. *Family Outing.* New York: Little, Brown and Co., 1998.

Brown, Mildred L. and Chloe Ann Rounsley. *True Selves: Understanding Transsexualism—For Families, Friends, Coworkers, and Helping Professionals.* San Francisco: Jossey-Bass Publishers, 1996.

Fone, Byrne. *Homophobia: A History.* New York: Metropolitan Books, 2000.

Gilbert, Susan. *A Field Guide to Boys and Girls.* New York: HarperCollins, 2000.

Greene, Beverly. "Ethnic-Minority Lesbians and Gay Men: Mental Health and Treatment Issues," *Journal of Consulting and Clinical Psychology,* 1994, Vol. 62, No. 2, 243–351.

Griffin, Carolyn Welch, Marlan J. Wirth and Arthur G. Wirth. *Beyond Acceptance: Parents of Lesbians and Gays Talk About Their Experiences.* New York: St. Martin's Press, 1996.

Hardin, Kimeron N., Ph.D. *The Gay and Lesbian Self-Esteem Book.* Oakland: New Harbinger Publications, 1999.

Hershberger, Scott, Neil W. Pilkington, and Anthony R. D'Augelli. "Predictors of Suicide Attempts Among Gay, Lesbian, and Bisexual Youth." *Journal of Adolescent Research,* Vol. 12, No. 4, Oct. 1997, 477–497.

Kimmel, Michael S. *The Gendered Society.* New York and Oxford: Oxford University Press, 2000.

Kirkham, Pat, editor. *The Gendered Object.* Manchester and New York: Manchester University Press, 1996.

Kroger, Jane. *Identity Development: Adolescence through Adulthood.* Thousand Oaks, CA: Sage Publications, 2000.

Maccoby, Eleanor. *The Two Sexes: Growing Up Apart, Coming Together.* Cambridge, MA: The Belknap Press of Harvard University, 1998.

Lipkin, Arthur. *Understanding Homosexuality, Changing Schools: A Text for Teachers, Counselors and Administrators.* Boulder, CO: Westview Press, 1998.

Maxym, Carol Ph.D. and Leslie B. York. *Teens in Turmoil: A Path to Change for Parents, Adolescents and Their Families.* New York: Viking, 2000.

Ponton, Lynn, M.D. *The Sex Lives of Teenagers.* New York: A Dutton Book, 2000.

Russell, Stephen I., Ph.D., and Kara Joyner, Ph.D. "Adolescent Sexual Orientation and Suicide Risk: Evidence from a National Study." *American Journal of Public Health*, August 2001, Vol. 91.

Ryan, Caitlin and Donna Futterman. *Lesbian and Gay Youth: Care and Counseling.* New York: Columbia University Press, 1998.

Savin-Williams, Ritch C. *Mom, Dad I'm Gay: How Families Negotiate Coming Out.* Washington, D.C.: American Psychological Association, 2001.

Shapiro, Patricia Gottlieb. *A Parent's Guide to Childhood and Adolescent Depression.* New York: Dell, 1994.

Yang, Alan S. *From Wrongs to Rights, Public Opinion on Gay and Lesbian Americans Toward Equality.* Washington, D.C.: NGLTF Policy Institute, 1999.

Yelland, Nicola, editor. *Gender in Early Childhood.* London, England: Routledge, 1998.

R E S O U R C E S

Recommended Books For Parents

Of General Interest

Aarons, Leroy. *Prayers for Bobby: A Mother's Coming to Terms With the Suicide of Her Gay Son.* San Francisco: Harper San Francisco, 1995.

Allen-Thompson, Pam and Di Allen-Thompson, LPCC. Ed. *The Beloved and 'Bent': Families Learning to Accept Lesbians and Gays.* Toledo, OH: Diversity Press, 1996.

Andrews, Nancy. *Family: A Portrait of Gay and Lesbian America.* San Francisco: Harper San Francisco, 1994.

Back, Gloria Guss. *Are You Still My Mother?* New York: Warner Books, 1985.

Bass, Ellen. *Free Your Mind.* New York: Harper Trade, 1996.

Bernstein, Robert. *Straight Parents, Gay Children: Inspiring Families to Live Honestly and with Greater Understanding.* Thunder Mouth Press, 1999.

Borhek, Mary V. *My Son Eric.* New York: The Pilgrim Press, 1979.

Buxton, Amity Pierce, Ph.D. *The Other Side of the Closet: The Coming-Out Crisis for Straight Spouses and Families.* New York: John Wiley and Sons, 1994.

Cantwell, Mary Ann. *Homosexuality: The Secret A Child Dare Not Tell.* Rafael Press, 1996.

Clark, Don, Ph.D. *Loving Someone Gay: Revised and Updated.* New York: Signet Books, 1987.

Clark, Patsy and Eloise Vaughn. *Keep Singing.* Los Angeles, New York: Alyson Books, 2001.

Degeneres, Betty. *Just A Mom.* CA: Advocate Books, 2001.

———. *Love, Ellen: A Mother/Daughter Journey.* New York: William Morrow and Co., 1999.

Dew, Robb Forman. *The Family Heart: A Memoir of When Our Son Came Out.* New York: Ballantine Books, 1995. Audio tape available from Simon & Schuster.

Fairchild, Betty and Nancy Hayward. *Now That You Know: What Every Parent Should Know About Homosexuality.* New York: Harcourt Brace, 1989.

Griffin, Carolyn Welch, Marlan J. Wirth and Arthur G. Wirth. *Beyond Acceptance: Parents of Lesbians and Gays Talk About Their Experiences.* New York: St. Martin's Press, 1996.

Herdt, Gilbert and Bruce Koff. *Something to Tell You—The Road that Families Travel When a Child is Gay.* New York: Columbia University Press, 2000.

Marcus, Eric. *Is It a Choice?: Answers to 300 of the Most Frequently Asked Questions About Gay and Lesbian People.* New York: HarperCollins, 1999.

Mastoon, Adam. *The Shared Heart: Portraits and Stories Celebrating Lesbian, Gay, and Bisexual Young People.* New York: HarperCollins, 2001.

McDougall, Bruce, Editor. *My Child is Gay.* Allen & Unwine, 1998.

Muller, Ann. *Parents Matter.* Tallahassee, FL: Naiad Press, 1987.

Owens, Robert E. *Queer Kids: The Challenges and Promise for Lesbian, Gay, and Bisexual Youth.* New York: Haworth Press, Inc., 1998.

Powers, Bob and Alan Ellis. *A Family and Friend's Guide to Sexual Orientation: Bridge the Divide between Gay and Straight.* New York and London: Routledge, 1996.

Rafkin, Louise. *Different Daughters: A Book by Mothers of Lesbians.* Pittsburgh, PA: Cleis Press, 1987.

Siegel, Laura and Nancy Lamkin Olson. *Out of the Closet—Into Our Hearts.* Leyland Publications, 2001.

Switzer, David K. *Coming Out as Parents: You and Your Homosexual Child.* Westminster/John Knox Press, 1996.

Tobias, Andrew (as John Reid). *The Best Little Boy in the World.* New York: Modern Library, 1998.

Woog, Dan. *Friends and Family: True Stories of Gay America's Straight Allies.* Alyson Publications, 1999.

On Gender Issues

Boyd-Franklin, Nancy and A. J. Franklin. *Boys Into Men: Raising Our African-American Teenage Sons.* New York: E.P. Dutton, 2000.

Pipher, Mary. *Reviving Ophelia: Saving the Selves of Adolescent Girls.* New York: Ballantine Books, 1994.

Pittman, Frank, M.D. *Man Enough.* New York: A Perigee Book, 1993.

Pollack, William S. *Real Boys: Rescuing Our Sons from the Myths of Boyhood.* Owl Books, 1999.

Kindlon, Dan, Ph.D. and Michael Thompson. *Raising Cain: Protecting the Emotional Lives of Boys.* New York: Ballantine Books, 1999.

On Talking with Teens about Sexuality

Harris, Robie. *It's Perfectly Normal: Growing Up, Changing Bodies, Sex and Sexual Health*. Cambridge, MA: Candlewick Press, 1994.

Madaras, Lynda with Area Madaras. *The What's Happening to My Body? Book for Boys—A Growing Up Guide for Parents and Sons*. New York: New Market Press, 1988.

Madaras, Lynda with Area Madaras. *The What's Happening to My Body? Book for Girls—A Growing Up Guide for Parents and Daughters*. New York: New Market Press, 1988.

Planned Parenthood Federation of America. *Talking About Sex—A Guide for Families* (video kit).

Slap, Gail, M.D. and Martha M. Jablow. *Teenage Health Care: The First Comprehensive Family Guide for the Preteen to Young Adult Years*. New York: Pocket Books, 1994.

On Religion and Homosexuality

Balka, Christie and Andy Rose, editors. *Twice Blessed: On Being Gay & Jewish*. Boston, MA: Beacon Press, 1989.

Bess, Rev. Howard H. *Pastor, I Am Gay*. Palmer Publishing Company, 1995.

Cromey, Robert Warren. *In God's Image; Christian Witness to the Need for Gay/Lesbian Equality in the Eyes of the Church*. San Francisco: Alamo Square Press, 1991.

Glaser, Chris. *Coming Out to God: Prayers for Lesbians and Gay Men, Their Families and Friends*. Westminster John Knox Press, 1991.

Hasbany, Richard, editor. *Homosexuality and Religion*. New York: Haworth Press, 1990.

Helminiak, Daniel A., Ph. D. *What the Bible Really Says About Homosexuality*. Alamo Square Press, May 2000.

Hilton, Bruce. *Can Homophobia Be Cured? Wrestling with Questions that Challenge the Church*. Abington Press, 1992.

McNeill, John. *Both Feet Firmly Planted in Midair: My Spiritual Journey*. Westminster John Knox Press, 1998.

Scanzoni, Letha and Virginia R. Mollenkott. *Is the Homosexual My Neighbor? A Positive Christian Response*. San Francisco: Harper San Francisco, 1994.

White, Rev. Mel. *Stranger at the Gate*. New York: Simon & Schuster, 1995.

On Transgenderism

Boenke, Mary, editor. *Trans Forming Families: Real Stories about Transgendered Loved Ones*. Walter Trook Publishing, 1999.

Brown, Mildred L. and Chloe Ann Rounsley. *True Selves: Understanding Transsexualism—For Families, Friends, Coworkers, and Helping Professionals*. San Francisco: Jossey-Bass Publishers, 1996.

Just Evelyn. *Mom, I Need to be a Girl*. The book, written by the mother of an MTF daughter, is available for $10.00 from Just Evelyn, 3707 Fifth Ave., #413, San Diego, CA 92103, or call 1-800-666-8158. Or contact http://www.justevelyn.com. The book's ISBN number is 0-9663272-09.

For additional reading suggestions, see GLSEN'S web site, www.glsen.org, or PFLAG's web site, www.pflag.org.

National Organizations

Gay, Lesbian and Straight Education Network (GLSEN) is a national organization with chapters in ninety cities that brings together students, teachers and community members to fight rigid gender roles, violence and anti-LGBT bias in schools. The web site, www.glsen.org, offers:

- the most current newspaper and magazine articles pertaining to anti-LGBT bias
- a resource library of articles and position papers
- help in locating a branch in your area

Parents, Friends and Families of Lesbians and Gays (PFLAG) is the premier organization for parents. Its web site, www.pflag.org, will help you:

- locate a chapter in your area
- get answers to questions parents commonly ask
- chat with other parents of LGBTQ youth

Lambda Legal Defense and Education Fund is the nation's oldest and largest legal organization working for the civil rights of lesbians, gay men and people with HIV/AIDS. For information on cases, briefs and decisions, consult its web site www.lambdalegal.org

National Youth Advocacy Coalition (NYAC) advocates for and with LGBTQ young people in an effort to end discrimination against them and to ensure their physical and emotional well-being. Its Bridges Project is the most comprehensive national clearinghouse for information and materials on issues affecting LGBTQ youth. Its web site is www.nyacyouth.org

Information on Advocating for Your Child

There are hundreds of resources to support you when you advocate for your child, depending on your particular situation and your needs. The following list will give you an idea of the range of resources available. These lists are constantly updated, so what's available now may change by the time you read this. Go to the web site listed below, search for the topic you are interested in and download the brochure. Following are some examples.

From GLSEN's web site, www.glsen.org:
• How to Start a Gay-Straight Alliance
• Working with School Boards
• Lobbying Tips
• Planning Your Visit to a State Official
• Sample Letters to a State Senator
• Hosting a Letter-Writing Party

From the American Civil Liberties Union web site, www.aclu.org:
• Tips on Meeting with Elected Officials
• Tips on Writing to Elected Officials
• Tips on Writing a Letter to the Editor
• Background Information of Lesbian and Gay Rights Legislation

Useful Booklets

• For a comprehensive and in-depth, systemic approach to solving problems in schools, consult "The GLSEN Workbook: A Developmental Model for Assessing, Describing and Improving Schools for Lesbian, Gay, Bisexual and Transgender (LGBT) People." Contact GLSEN at (212) 727-0135 for a copy.

• "Taking the Offensive in the Struggle Against Anti-Gay Abuse in Public Schools: Improving School Policies and State Laws." Contact Lambda Legal Defense and Education Fund National Headquarters at (212) 809-8585 for a copy.

• "Stopping Anti-Gay Abuse of Students in Public Schools: A Legal perspective." Contact Lambda Legal Defense and Education Fund National Headquarters at (212) 809-8585 for a copy.

To get a copy of your state policies, go to the following web sites:
- www.glsen.org
- www.lambdalegal.org
- www.aclu.org

For the most up-to-date information on current laws and legislation, consult the following web sites:
- Lambda Legal Defense and Education Fund: www.lambdalegal.org
- American Civil Liberties Union: www.aclu.org
- The National Center for Lesbian Rights: www.nclrights.org
- Gay and Lesbian Advocates and Defenders: www.glad.org

Web Sites

For Information on Talking with Your Child about Sexual Issues
- www.siecus.org—A site dedicated to promoting communication and education about sex with special tips for parents that are honest, accurate and developmentally appropriate.
- www.talkingwithkids.org—A resource for parents on talking with kids about a variety of tough issues, including sex.
- www.youthresource.com—A web site created by and for LGBTQ young people from thirteen to twenty-four years old. It takes a holistic approach to sexual health by offering support, community resources and peer-to-peer education about health, advocacy, community and other issues.

For LGBT Youth that May Be of Interest to Parents
- www.outproud.org—A national coalition for LGBT youth with links to school resources library, coming out stories, and local sources of support and friendship
- www.youth.org—a service run by volunteers to help LGBT youth express themselves, feel supported and interact with others who have accepted their sexuality. This site is especially good for questioning youth. It also has links to other sites for LGBT youth.
- www.planetout.com—a general web site for LGBTQ people offering information on news and politics, money and careers,

entertainment, travel and personal ads and chat rooms. It has special links for youth.

- www.alliesproject.org—This web site is sponsored by the Straight Allies Project, which tries to engage straight Americans in the struggle for LGBT equality.
- www.mogenic.com—the world's number one web site for LGBT youth of color.

Of Faith-Based Groups Where Parents Can Meet Others Who Have Reconciled Their Religious Beliefs with LGBT Issues

- www.dignityusa.org (Catholics)
- www.gaychristian.net
- www.integrityusa.org (Episcopalians)
- www.soulforce.org
- www.interfaithalliance.org
- www.ufmcc.com
- www.GayJews.org (Orthodox Jews)

For Parents of Transgendered Youth

National referral resources to find a gender therapist or to obtain other information on transgender issues:

- Renaissance Transgender Association at www.ren.org or (610) 975-9119
- Gender Education & Advocacy (GEA) at www.gender.org (no phone)
- The International Foundation for Gender Education (IFGE) at www.ifge.org or (781) 899-2212. It publishes an excellent quarterly magazine that contains a detailed resource guide listing community organizations and professionals in the field.
- Harry Benjamin International Gender Dysphoria Association (HBIGDA) at www.HBIGDA.org or (415) 322-2335. HBIGDA is a professional organization, not designed to serve the public. There is a lot of information at the HBIGDA web site, though, including the Standards of Care and the International Journal of Transgenderism, which contains many useful articles for professionals. You may want to pass this resource along to any medical care providers who work with your family and who are not already familiar with transgender medicine.

- www.gendertalk.com is a web site with information on trans issues with connections to the leading talk radio program on gender issues, a calendar of events and other links.

For Transgendered Youth

1. Youth Resource's Trans*topic Pages http://www.youth
resource.com/feat/trans/index.html
2. Mermaids (from the UK) http://www.mermaids.freeuk.com
3. The AntiJen Pages http://www.antijen.org
4. TransBoy Resource Network http://www.geocities.
com/WestHollywood/Park/6484

For Parents and Youth of Color

- Youth Resource—www.youthresource.com—a web site created by and for LGBTQ young people from thirteen to twenty-four years old offering support, community, resources and peer-to-peer education about health, advocacy, community and other issues. It has several links for young men and women of color.
- The Black Stripe—www.blackstripe.com—a web site for LGBT African Americans
- Gay Asian Pacific Alliance (GAPA)—www.gapa.org—a web site for Asian Pacific LGBT people
- National Latino/a Lesbian, Gay, Bisexual and Transgender Organization (LLEGO)—www.llego.org—a web site for Latino/a LGBT individuals
- Trikone—www.trikone.org—a web site for LGBT South Asians
- The top three web sites for Native Americans:
  www.homestead.com/twospiritsociety/tss1.html
  www.nnaapc.org/tsv/tsv01.html
  www.temenos.net/poc/twospirit/

Referral Sources for Therapists Who Work with LGBTQ Youth

- Contact the National Association of Social Workers (NASW) for a list of its gay and lesbian caucuses. (800) 227-3590.
- Contact the American Psychological Association through its national office in Washington, D.C., for a local referral. (800) 259-2666.

PFLAG Recommended Videos

• "Always My Kid: A Family Guide to Understanding Homosexuality" (1994, 74 minutes) Triangle Video Productions, 550 Westcott, Suite 400, Houston, Texas 77007; (713) 869-4477; Fax: (713) 861-1577.

• "Straight From The Heart: Stories Of Parents' Journeys To a New Understanding of Their Lesbian and Gay Children" (1994, 26 minutes) Dee Mosbacher, producer. Motivational Media, 8430 Santa Monica Blvd., Los Angeles, CA 90069; (800) 848-2707.

• "Queer Son: Family Journeys To Understanding and Love" (1994, 48 minutes) Vickie Seitchik, 19 Jackson Street, Cape May, NJ 08204; (212) 929-4199.

Additional Videos

All the following are available from PFLAG Denver. Contact: Tim Wilson, P.O. Box 18901, Denver, CO 80218-0901; (303) 573-5861; fax (303) 573-3949.

• "Accepting Your Gay or Lesbian Child"—90-minute audio cassette featuring six parents who overcame their prejudices about homosexuality. ($11.00)

• "An Unexpected Journey"—This national-award-winning 30-minute video focuses on the coming out process for gays and lesbians and their parents' acceptance. ($30.00)

• "When Your Child Comes Out To You"—Video in six workshop sessions (1 hr. 40 min. total) produced by Metropolitan Community Church of Boulder; workshop is led by the first heterosexual minister ordained by the International Fellowship of MCC.

Best Gay Youth Movies

We put out a call over GLSEN's email listserv to ask students what movies they'd recommend. Here were some of their recommendations and thoughts, with the caveat that parents should consider the ratings attached by the Motion Picture Association of America to these films and make their own decisions about how appropriate they are:

Beautiful Thing: This film depicts two young boys from different backgrounds coming to terms with being gay and finding love in a working-class London neighborhood.

Billy Elliot: A moving Academy Award–nominated film about a young boy who battles gender- and sexual-orientation stereotypes to pursue his dream of being a ballet dancer in a working-class English community.

Boys Don't Cry: "First movie I saw about transsexual issues," writes one student. Based on a true story, *Boys* contains vivid depictions of violence. Hillary Swank won an Academy Award for her portrayal of Brandon Teena, an FTM transgender person who was killed in Nebraska in the late nineties.

De Colores: Available in both English and Spanish, this film covers the "multiple identities" aspect of being Latina/o and LGBT. Parents and their sons/daughters talk about coming out and the issues they have to face as Latino parents.

Edge of Seventeen: Set in Ohio during the eighties, this film depicts a young man's coming-out story in a way that is true to the "out," then "in," then "out" process many teens go through.

Get Real: Set in England, this movie tells the story of Steven, sixteen, who knows that he's gay. Life changes for him when he locks eyes on John, the school's handsome super-jock. The two are attracted to each other, but John's fears threaten to tear apart their tentative relationship. One student writes that "this is a good movie for students and parents looking to understand what coming out is really like."

The Incredibly True Adventure of Two Girls in Love: This film tells the story of two teenage girls coming to terms with their lesbian identities and finding love.

Kissing Jessica Stein: A student writes that she found it "very interesting because it was about a woman who tries lesbianism just out of curiosity, and ends up realizing that she is bisexual. It depicts such a nonstereotypical approach with great characters and a wonderful script. Anyone would enjoy this movie."

Ma Vie En Rose (My Life in Pink): A French film in which a family comes to terms with their grade schooler's "coming out" as transgender.

MTV True Life: I'm Coming Out: A documentary in which four young people and their families negotiate the coming out process with a variety of reactions and results—all filmed live on camera.

The Truth About Jane: Based on a true story. Jane's mom assumes her popular daughter is just like every other fifteen-year-old girl. Then Jane meets Taylor and falls madly in love with her. Suddenly, everyone is trying to figure out how to cope with the realization that Jane is a lesbian.

Trevor: An Academy Award–winning short film about a junior high boy who learns it is OK to be both gay *and* obsessed with Diana Ross.

INDEX

ACLU, state listing of discrimination laws, 245; suit against Orangeview Junior High School Library, 253

African American LGBTQ teens. *See* LGBTQ youth of color

alcohol. *See* substance abuse

Alexander the Great, 73

American Beauty (film), 45

American culture: bias, for heterosexuality, 5–8, 66–67; educating yourself about your child's world, 52–55; gender stereotypes, 7–8, 65–66, 67–70; history of anti-LGBT bias, 72–75; hostility and psychological problems in homosexuals, 77; questioning teens and, 198–99; television or video, what to do if something disturbs you, 53–54; tolerance for homosexuality, 74–75

American Psychological Association (APA): referrals, 274; removal of homosexuality as an illness from *Diagnostic and Statistical Manual*, 77; on sexual orientation, 76, 77

ANRED (Anorexia Nervosa and Related Eating Disorders, Inc.), 266

APICHA (Asian Pacific Islander Coalition HIV Association), 235

Barrios, Jarret, 232

Bartle, Nathalie, 32

bigotry against LGBT youth, 99–100; bullies and bigots, who they are, 104–6; four signs your child is being bullied, 106; name-calling, 101–2, 240–41; physical assaults, 203; preparing your child to handle school harassment, 106–10; shunning and ostracism, 100–101; statistics, 100; stopping the cycle,

106; threats of violence, 102–3; three-step process for self-protection, 108–10. *See also* laws and legal protection for your child

bisexual youth: model for coming out, 136–39; myths about, 78–79, 137; suggestions for parents, 138–39

Bono, Chastity, 23, 34, 141

Bowie, David, 163

Boy George, 163

Boys Don't Cry (film), 186

Buffy the Vampire Slayer (TV series), 43, 52

bullying, 104–6; three-step process for self-protection, 108–10; when your harassed child comes home, 110–13. *See also* bigotry against LGBT youth

Cannibals and Christians (Mailer), 82–83

Carragher, Danny, 114

Cho, Margaret, 231

Cohn, Roy, 74

coming out, 11; admission and retraction of statement, 2; blending parents' and child's process, 128–29; earlier age of, 46–47; fears of, 121, 136, 294; four ways to prepare your child to come out to straight friends, 97–98; Mega-Model for accepting and integrating identity, 122–24; parental acceptance, broadening of by telling others, 149–54; parent's process, 124–30, 135–36; model for bisexual youth, 136–39; model for gay and lesbian youth, 122, 134–36; parental breaking the ice, 130–33; siblings' process, 144–49; to straight friends, 95–98; subsequent conversations about, 160–61;

ABOUT THE AUTHORS

KEVIN JENNINGS is cofounder and executive director of the Gay, Lesbian and Straight Education Network (GLSEN), which has ninety chapters nationwide. A New Yorker, he was named to *Newsweek*'s "Century Club" as one of 100 people to watch in the new century.

PATRICIA GOTTLIEB SHAPIRO, M.S.W., is the author of five nonfiction books including *A Parent's Guide to Childhood and Adolescent Depression*. She lives in Santa Fe, New Mexico.